bedwetting

A treatment manual for professional staff

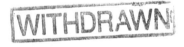

Bedwetting *A treatment manual for professional staff*

J. Bollard PhD — *Department of Psychiatry*
Adelaide Children's Hospital Inc.
Adelaide, South Australia

and

T. Nettelbeck PhD — *Department of Psychology*
University of Adelaide
Adelaide, South Australia

 Chapman and Hall   *London   New York*

First published in 1989 by Chapman and Hall Ltd
11 New Fetter Lane, London EC4P 4EE

© 1989 Jeff Bollard and Ted Nettelbeck

Typeset in 10½/12pt Sabon by Mayhew Typesetting, Bristol

Printed in Great Britain by St Edmundsbury Press,
Bury St. Edmunds, Suffolk

ISBN 0 412 32520 9

British Library Cataloguing in Publication Data

Bollard, J. (Jeffrey), 1949–
  Bedwetting.
  1. Children. Enuresis. Prevention
  I. Title II. Nettelbeck, Ted, 1936–
  618.92' 63
  ISBN 0–412–32520–9

Contents

Preface

In our experience as psychologists, a major childhood problem today concerns the large numbers of children who do not exercise appropriate control of the bladder during sleep, and there seems little reason to doubt that this has always been so. According to Glicklich's (1951) historical account of enuresis, bedwetting was considered to be of sufficient importance to warrant attention in European medical textbooks as early as the sixteenth century. Early interest in bedwetting focused on treatment rather than causation and, probably as a result of confusion about the nature and aetiology of the problem, a very wide range of therapeutic procedures were employed. It was common during the middle ages to require enuretic children to swallow a variety of 'medicines', such as the ground cerebrum of a hare, the pulverized bladder of a young breeding sow, the lung of a young goat, the flesh of a ground hedgehog, the inside skin of the stomach of hens and the urine of spayed swine. Punishment also featured heavily in the prescriptions followed in earlier times, this ranging from beating the enuretic child to public ridicule, severe threats and even the administration of blisters to the sacrum. The middle ages were also times of strong religious beliefs so that, not surprisingly, the treatment of enuresis frequently included prayer and ceremonies, like requiring the enuretic child to wear a white smock at baptism. Very severe, cruel punishment following incontinence is certainly less common today, although such instances are, unhappily, reported from time to time (Schaefer, 1979). It is, moreover, still the case that spanking is not an infrequent parental response to a wet bed, although all the evidence confirms that punishment in this form is unlikely to alleviate the problem.

Attention to causal theories of enuresis becomes much more obvious in the medical literature of the nineteenth century and, interestingly, the basis of many modern-day theories can be found in these writings. For example, it was noted at this time that there seems to be a tendency for the disorder to recur among the children of past bedwetters, and that there appears to be an association between deep sleep and enuresis. Other explanations focused on pathology of the musculature within the bladder and on abnormality of the neurological pathways involved in bladder control. Poor motivation on the part of the child and poor training by the child's parent or caregiver were also considered in the nineteenth century to be likely to result in faulty habits and were therefore regarded as the primary aetiological factors underlying bedwetting.

By the close of the nineteenth century enuresis was a widely recognized disorder, commanding considerable space in the textbooks of the day. However, disagreement about the causes and treatment of the problem persisted. This confusion is reflected in the wide array of poorly founded and bizarre and sometimes contradictory curative measures commonly practised during the first half of the twentieth century. These procedures included advice like raising the head of the bed (or raising the foot of the bed), requiring the enuretic child to sleep on its back (or sleep on its tummy), sleeping on a bed of cotton reels, special diets, a wide range of tonic drugs, various gadgets to prevent urine leaving the urethra, electric shock to the genitals in response to wetting accidents and a number of surgical procedures including circumcision. It also became common practice in the early part of the twentieth century to advise parents against any form of therapy, this recommendation being motivated by the belief that the best 'cure' was simply to allow the child to outgrow the disorder. In connection with this advice it was sometimes suggested that spontaneous remission of bedwetting symptoms occurred in seven year cycles; i.e. it was suggested that children typically outgrew the problem at 7 years of age, or at 14 or 21 years of age.

The forerunner to the modern urine-alarm device for the

treatment of bedwetting dates from the beginning of the twentieth century, although there had been earlier suggestions for contrivances using electricity which proved to be too cumbersome or impractical for other reasons. In 1904 Pfaundler devised an apparatus which, when placed in the beds of children living in a state institution, emitted an auditory signal in response to bedwetting episodes. The original intention of this arrangement was merely to alert an attendant that the child had urinated but in doing so it was accidentally discovered that this alarm system resulted in the arrest of bedwetting episodes in many of the children. This apparatus was subsequently refined by psychologists and the urine-alarm systems widely employed today differ from the Pfaundler equipment only in terms of more recent advances in electronics.

Debate about the nature and aetiology of enuresis has continued into the latter half of the twentieth century. However, there is now a growing consensus of opinion that, for the majority of enuretic children, the problem represents a learning or habit deficiency. In addition, it is widely recognized that current treatment procedures are highly effective in at least about 80% of all such cases in arresting the problem, as will be shown in subsequent sections of this book. In this manual we have set out what is currently known about the cause and treatment of nocturnal enuresis in children who have essentially normal intelligence. In our discussion of the considerable body of research literature that is now available on this topic we have tried to minimize dependence on supporting references, while at the same time providing sufficient details to permit a reader to follow up technical considerations, should he or she wish to do so. Detailed accounts of relevant research, together with extensive bibliographies on the topic, are provided by Kolvin *et al.* (1973), Sorotzkin (1984), Butler (1987) and by Bollard and Nettelbeck (in press). A reader interested in the treatment of enuresis among intellectually disabled children should refer to Azrin *et al.* (1973) and to Bettison (1986). For information about the management of day-time wetting, which arguably has a different morphology to night-time bedwetting, the reader is directed to Bettison (1979), to Azrin and Foxx (1974) and to Smith and Smith (1987). The book by Smith and Smith (1987) is recommended as essential reading for anyone interested in the normal development of continence and the broad spectrum of incontinence problems. While the major thrust of the Smith and Smith book concerns the development of day-time urinary continence and the application of this information to the management of day-time urinary incontinence, there is a comprehensive chapter on bedwetting. The main theoretical framework for treatment of incontinence is based on a combination of developmental and operant views. Considerable attention is also given to problems of encopresis, incontinence in adults and mentally retarded people, and loss of continence associated with dementia. The practitioner will find particularly useful the chapter on training guidelines; this is intended for diurnal enuresis but many of the principles and strategies outlined are also directly applicable to bedwetting. Finally, Mandelstam (1986) provides a wide-ranging discussion of topics relating to the mechanisms and management of urinary incontinence among adults, including a number of gynaecological and neurological conditions, areas of disability, and focusing particularly on the problems of elderly people. Mandelstam's book also includes a well-developed glossary of technical terminology and an account of a range of aids to the treatment of incontinence, other than the bedwetting alarm, which are available in the United Kingdom.

We wish to record our thanks to Judy Fallon and Cynthia Voet (University of Adelaide) and Colleen Lloyd (Adelaide Children's Hospital) for their assistance in the preparation of the figures, and to Kathryn Tolhurst, Sophie Tzamtzidis, and Carol McCulloch, word processor operators and secretaries in the Department of Psychology, University of Adelaide, for their good natured patience and efficiency when typing the manuscript.

1
Theory and treatment

1.1 Introduction, definition and incidence

The term **enuresis** is commonly used to refer to persistent
childhood bedwetting, which occurs in the absence of any
discernible neurological or urological pathology, and which
continues beyond an age by which most children, without the
need for special attention, have gained normal control over
functioning of the bladder. Strictly speaking, a distinction
should be made between the passing of urine (micturition) at
night during sleep (nocturnal enuresis) and involuntary
wetting that occurs during the day when the child is awake
(diurnal enuresis); and nor is enuresis restricted only to
childhood. However, the tendency of some children, older
than about three to five years of age, to continue to wet the
bed frequently, is a much more common problem than either
day-time wetting among children or nocturnal enuresis
among adults; approximately 80% of enuretic children wet
only at night, while incidence among adults probably does
not exceed 1%. For these reasons, then, it is quite common
to use enuresis for problem childhood bedwetting but to
provide more detailed descriptions when referring to other
enuretic problems.

There is no particular age by which the normal child will
achieve control of micturition while asleep. A small number
of children (perhaps as many as 6–8% according to some
estimates) actually become permanently dry at night before
one year of age and, according to evidence on physiological
maturation, most children are capable of establishing such
control by about three to four years of age. In fact, however,
cultural expectations about the development of continence at
night vary widely. For example, recent epidemiological data

for three-year-old children in an outer London (UK) borough have suggested reliably lower rates of bedwetting among British children of Asian origin, when compared with other British children (Weir, 1982). As another example, the problem of nocturnal enuresis, as indicated by the numbers of parents seeking treatment for their children, appears to be more prevalent in the USA and in Australia than in the UK or in Sweden. The problem has also sometimes been reported more frequently among children from working-class homes than among children of middle-class parents, although Weir's recent study involving 705 three-year-olds found no association between bedwetting and social class or housing conditions.

There are substantial difficulties in estimating the prevalence of problem bedwetting, even in technologically advanced countries, although reliable information about general population trends based on prevalence in various British, European, Australian and United States locations has been available for about 30 years. De Jonge (1973) has surveyed this work and has included a comprehensive summary of epidemiological research up to that time. Studies of morbidity risk, defined as the presence of enuresis at some time beyond a specified age (for example three years of age) are rare and most epidemiological research has been concerned with incidence – that is, the percentage of cases of active enuresis identified at the time of the investigation. A major recent Dutch survey (Verhulst et al., 1985), based on a sample of more than 2000 children aged from 4 to 16 years, has substantially confirmed incidence findings in the earlier studies. Although different studies have reported widely different estimates of the proportions of children described as being enuretic at various ages, the overall incidence of bedwetting is known to decrease rapidly and steadily from infancy, with a marked decline in prevalence beyond ages six to eight years and with bedwetting becoming rare from about twelve years of age. However, a small proportion of individuals continue to wet the bed regularly as adolescents and some even continue bedwetting into adulthood. Another important general finding is that bedwetting is somewhat more frequent in boys than among girls up until the age of about eleven years, perhaps because of sex-linked differences in rate of maturation.

Individual patterns in the incidence of bedwetting vary one from another, with some children wetting the bed several times each night, others wetting only occasionally, and still others wetting sporadically but heavily. Also, there is no clear agreement among researchers in the field about the minimum frequency of bedwetting before a child should be regarded as enuretic; thus, some researchers have regarded an incidence of at least one wet bed per month as sufficient evidence for the existence of a problem requiring treatment, while others have required at least two wet nights per week. The definition currently recommended by the American Psychiatric Association (1980) in its third edition of the *Diagnostic and Statistical Manual of Mental Disorders* (DSM III), requires an incidence of at least two wetting episodes a month for children between the ages of five and six years, and once a month for older children. Methods of investigation have varied with different surveys and the populations sampled have varied widely. Furthermore, some experts consider that there are actually two types of nocturnal enuresis; a primary form, usually assumed to be the consequence of maturational delay and/or faulty learning, and lifelong to that point in time, so that the child has never achieved complete control over night-time micturition; and a secondary or acquired type which is characterized by a previous significant period of nocturnal continence (usually achieved for more than six months) but with this then being followed by a return to a pattern of regular night-time wetting. It has sometimes been suggested that secondary enuresis is more likely to be accompanied by evidence of psychological stress or of some organic pathology. To this time at least, however, there is little reliable evidence that this distinction has significance for prognosis, since most cases of enuresis categorized as primary or secondary appear to respond to treatment in essentially the same way. None the less, it is also our experience that where the onset of bedwetting can plausibly be associated with identifiable stressful circumstances and/or observed recent changes in the child's general demeanour, then it is necessary first to attempt to address such issues before proceeding with treatment. In other words, it remains our belief that, although strong empirical evidence in support of this distinction is not available, it often seems to be the case that the distinction between primary and secondary forms of enuresis can be of practical use.

Despite problems like these when attempting to estimate prevalence, studies employing a criterion of at least one wet night per month have suggested several important trends with respect to the incidence of bedwetting. Thus, at least in Western European/North American cultures, about 7% of children actually achieve complete nocturnal continence by the time that they reach their first birthday. The incidence of bedwetting drops rapidly over the next two years, with different epidemiological studies finding that between about 50–70% of three-year-olds in these cultures are continent. Thereafter the residual number of bedwetters continues to decline but much less markedly. About 10–15% of five-year-olds continue to wet the bed regularly, with incidence falling to about 5–6% for ten-year-olds, 2–3% for teenagers and, thereafter, an apparently steady 1% of cases continuing on throughout adulthood. This trend is illustrated in Figure 1.1. Whether the decreasing trend seen in this figure is better represented as the smooth function drawn, following Lovibond (1964), or by a step-function, as implied by the data points included in the figure, cannot be determined reliably at this time. One finds considerable variation in incidence across the various studies yet available, particularly between the ages of four and eleven years, for which most data are available. The trend shown has been estimated from studies surveyed by De Jonge (1973; including his Addendum) and from the recent large-scale study by Verhulst et al. (1985) in the Netherlands. A general, widespread finding, across the full age range, is that incidence is consistently somewhat higher among males than females, the ratio being approximately 3:2. These estimates for the incidence of bedwetting have now been confirmed for several different countries at

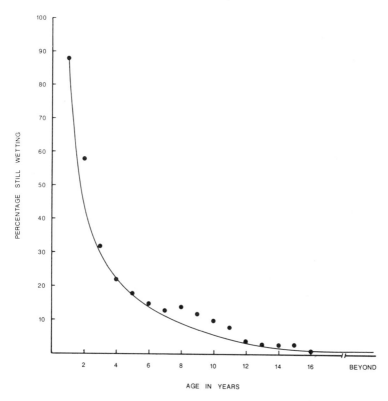

Figure 1.1 The incidence of bedwetting, expressed in percentages, at different ages. Data points represent arithmetic means, estimated from summary data published by De Jonge (1973) and Verhulst *et al.* (1985).

different levels of economic development and may be regarded as representative. A point worth emphasizing here is that, while the percentages of children who wet the bed regularly beyond the ages of 7–10 years may not seem at first to be unduly pronounced, the actual numbers of cases involved at any point in time will be very large indeed. As a consequence, from a management perspective the scale of the problem is vast, and particularly so in highly urbanized cultures where large numbers of children are congregated in densely populated areas. Although it is not invariably so, in our experience most children beyond the age of seven who wet the bed do wish to become dry, the most frequent reason given being that incontinence severely limits their ability to sleep away from home, at a friend's house or on a school trip. Among parents, major concerns expressed refer to the emotional well-being and adequate social activities of the child, although a significant proportion of mothers are also anxious to reduce the burden of having to clean up after an enuretic child.

The relatively high rate at which incidence for being dry at night emerges between the ages of about one to four years, compared to lower rates either before or following these years (among those children still wetting the bed), has suggested the possibility that mechanisms responsible for controlling micturition normally mature during this period. Thus, MacKeith *et al.* (1973) have speculated about a 'sensitive' or optimal period, not dependent upon learning or training, during which dryness is destined to emerge unless stress or illness or unrealistic, restrictive toilet training interferes.

1.2 The physiology of micturition

THE MECHANISM OF MICTURITION

As illustrated in Figure 1.2, the urinary bladder comprises two principal parts: (1) the detrusor muscle in the main body of the organ, and (2) the trigone. The detrusor is a smooth, involuntary muscle forming the wall to the bladder. The trigone is a muscular mass near the mouth of the bladder through which pass two tubes, termed ureters, which convey urine from each kidney to the bladder, and the canal through which urine is discharged, called the urethra. The trigonal muscle embraces a smaller muscle, called the internal sphincter, which acts to open and close the bladder at this location. Below this the urethra passes through another muscle, the external sphincter of the bladder.

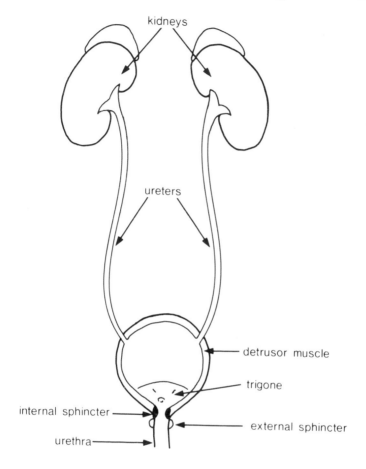

Figure 1.2 The urinary bladder and its collecting system.

Although the act of micturition is described here as a relatively simple reflex, it is actually a very complex response resulting from an integrated chain of reflexes. As urine passes through the ureters it accumulates in the bladder and muscle tone in the detrusor is repeatedly adjusted to allow larger volumes of urine to be stored, with little increase in the internal pressure. A normal adult can, in fact, store up to about 200 ml of urine before the pressure within the bladder increases significantly. However, with further distension beyond this volume, nervous impulses arise from the stimulation of the sensory end organs in the bladder wall and these impulses trigger reflex micturition. This action involves strong rhythmical contractions of the detrusor muscle, relaxation of the internal sphincter followed by relaxation of the external sphincter and, ultimately, the passing of urine.

THE DEVELOPMENT OF BLADDER CONTROL

Detailed accounts of the development of bladder control are provided by Muellner (1960a, 1960b), Yates (1975) and Smith and Smith (1987). Maturation of the parasympathetic nervous system ensures that most infants between one and two years of age will gradually achieve an improved awareness of increasing bladder tension as the bladder fills. The child's initially small functional bladder capacity is consequently increased and the incidence of reflex voiding in response to bladder distension becomes less frequent. By three years of age most children have learned to tense the perineal muscles in the crutch, thereby raising the bladder neck and tightening the internal sphincter, so that urine in the full bladder can be retained for a considerable time. With increasing functional bladder capacity the frequency of voiding drops and a larger volume is passed. By between three and four years of age most children have achieved the ability to start the urine flow from a full bladder, by pushing down of the thoracic wall and tightening the abdominal muscles at the same time. By about four years of age most children can also stop the urinary stream at will. For the achievement of nocturnal continence it is assumed that the child learns to transfer inhibitory control over micturition to locations in the cortex which develop the capability to detect detrusor muscle contractions and inhibit sphincter relaxation. In this way, urine is either retained throughout the hours of sleep or, when bladder tension is excessive, the child wakes up. In most cases, this level of control is achieved, apart from very occasional lapses, by about three to four years of age. This is a consequence of the increasing volume of fluid which the bladder can store without evacuating contractions occurring, together with a reduced level of urine production during sleep. On those occasions during sleep when pressure in the bladder exceeds the limits of compensatory adjustment in the detrusor muscle, feedback stimulation from the filling bladder wakes the child before the micturitional reflex is triggered. In most cases full continence will develop by about six years of age, by which time the ability to start urination at almost any degree of bladder filling has been mastered and the child finally learns to initiate micturition reliably only in appropriate places.

There is not widespread agreement about a recommended age beyond which it is preferable to initiate treatment for bedwetting. Most experts appear not to favour a treatment programme if the child is younger than about five years of age, the age incorporated within the DSM III definition, although others have argued for earlier intervention, perhaps as young as three years old. Still another point of view emphasizes family and social considerations, rather than any particular age, suggesting that a decision to begin treatment should depend upon the extent to which bedwetting is disrupting the normal social and emotional development of the child.

PATHOPHYSIOLOGY OF THE GENITO-URINARY SYSTEM

Cases of enuresis caused by organic disease are rare, even among older children, probably constituting no more than about 5% of the total enuretic population. In fact, even among individuals with an infection of the urinary tract, the incidence of enuresis is still not especially high, although enuresis does occur in association with urinary tract infections. It may, for example, be secondary to the excessive production of urine (polyuria) caused by diabetes mellitus, diabetes insipidus or renal tubular defects. Also, the likelihood of an association between night-time bedwetting and organic disease is increased if diurnal enuresis is also present. However, curing an infection of the urinary tract has not generally been found to eradicate bedwetting and there is no evidence to suggest that organic pathology causes bedwetting in other than a relatively very small number of cases. None the less, every child identified as requiring treatment for nocturnal enuresis must first be examined by a medical practitioner, so as to exclude an explanation in terms of some organic disorder. Incontinence may be associated with spina bifida or with other neurological disorders like nocturnal epilepsy. Neuropathic bladders that never fill because of poor resistance at the urethra are almost always associated with other somatic neurological signs, such as perineal anaesthesia, and absent or poor rectal tone, impaired bowel control, and disturbances in gait. If one ureter is located in an abnormal position, this may produce dribbling incontinence, despite normal micturition at regular intervals; similarly, obstruction of the bladder outlet or urethra may result in overflow incontinence.

1.3 Theories of enuresis and associated methods for treatment

Not surprisingly, the problem of nocturnal enuresis in childhood has been recognized since ancient times and the literature on the subject therefore has an extensive history, as outlined briefly in the Preface to this book. Many different explanations about the nature and cause of nocturnal enuresis have been put forward, with different recommendations about treatment reflecting different theoretical positions. However, in broad terms, modern theoretical explanations and associated treatments fall into three categories: psychodynamic theories, which recommend treatment by psychotherapy; physiological theories associated with some form of medical intervention; and behavioural theories and treatments. Each of these categories is discussed in turn in the sections that follow.

PSYCHODYNAMIC THEORIES AND TREATMENT

The essential idea underlying the general psychodynamic position is that enuresis is only an outward manifestation of some underlying state of emotional tension or instability. Where couched in psychoanalytical terminology, like a substitution for repressed sexual drive, or the result of a repressed Oedipal complex, a theory of this kind remains essentially untestable, with any evidence necessarily confined to clinical impressions. However, another kind of psychodynamic theory characterizes enuresis as a consequence of unresolved conflict, for example, between a child and the parents, or involving other persons significant in the child's life. Expressed in these terms, theories of this kind are open to empirical investigation, since they predict that a substantially greater degree of anxiety and emotional maladjustment should be found among a representative sample of enuretic children than in a comparable group of nonenuretics matched for age, IQ, educational level, socio-economic status and other variables that have been found to be associated with the incidence of enuresis.

It is certainly the case that a majority of investigations into this hypothesis have found some degree of association between enuresis and evidence for emotional or behavioural disorders (Shaffer, 1973; Sorotzkin, 1984). This general finding is therefore, to some extent, at odds with the usual behavioural position, which rejects an association between enuresis and psychological disturbance. Despite considerable research, however, there is not clear evidence to support this type of psychodynamic theory as a general proposition. One problem is simply that it is excessively difficult to evaluate emotional health in children. Another is that, although general population surveys such as the Reykjavik, Iceland survey (Bjornsson, 1973), the Isle of Wight investigation (Rutter *et al.*, 1973) and the National Child Development study (Essen and Peckham, 1976) have found some evidence of a higher than expected incidence of enuresis among children with psychological disorders (particularly those children with the common neurotic and conduct disorders) these surveys have also emphasized that most enuretic children are actually well adjusted and free from other problems affecting their behaviour. In other words, the majority of enuretic children have not been found to be discernably different from nonenuretic children in this regard. Wier's 1982 London study, referred to in section 1.1, found no associations between bedwetting and several measures of stress due to social, emotional or health problems, although the children in this study were three-year-olds and the effects of stress variables might be more obvious at later ages. None the less, comparative studies of the personalities of enuretics and nonenuretics have also failed to find clear support for the psychodynamic position (Lovibond, 1964; Collins, 1973). Although psychological disorders are sometimes accompanied by either or both night-time and day-time urinary incontinence, even so, the majority of enuretic children do not display behavioural difficulties other than bedwetting. Thus, while it is the case that some instances of enuresis appear to be related directly to traumatic circumstances in childhood, it may be more useful to regard both the enuresis and the stress experienced as reactive to specific environmental circumstances. These might involve perhaps separation from the mother, the loss of a parent or inadequate care on the part of the parents, or some other form of stress at home or at school. However, it remains the case that no such explanation can be found to apply among the great majority of chronic bedwetters.

Furthermore, even if an enuretic child does show signs of emotional disturbance, this disturbance is not necessarily the cause of the enuresis but may, instead, be the consequence of the enuresis itself. Thus, Lovibond (1964) has pointed out that persistent enuresis can result in important limitations in the child's social life that could upset the child – like feeling that one cannot stay overnight at a friend's house for fear of having an embarrassing accident. It is clear then that, before concluding that some postulated stress or conflict has resulted in the enuresis, it must be shown that an emotional disturbance has preceded or coincided with the onset of acquired enuresis; or, in the case of primary enuresis, such emotional instability should have been evident at a time when the child would normally have been becoming dry. To date, however, we are not aware of any evidence that would clearly support this position.

A second point made by theorists with a psychodynamic orientation is consistent with psychoanalytic views about symptom substitution. The psychodynamic position has generally been that, simply to treat the symptom itself is both futile and undesirable, since this treatment does not deal with the emotional disturbance assumed to underlie poor control over continence. Thus, the untreated emotional disturbance is held to remain the real problem. Indeed, some psychoanalytic theorists have insisted that it can be dangerous to eliminate enuresis directly, since underlying anxieties may be exacerbated by this intervention, which may then serve to produce some other serious disturbance. Lovibond (1964) has addressed such issues at length, arguing strongly that the eradication of bedwetting is beneficial to overall psychological health. This view is consistent with his opinion that prolonged enuresis may actually result in psychological disturbance, and his position is supported by research evidence. Thus, the elimination of nocturnal enuresis following direct treatment has been shown to be, at the very least, psychologically benign; and more often beneficial, when compared with alternative forms of treatment (Shaffer, 1973; Sacks et al., 1974; Dische, et al., 1983). Even in cases where the direct treatment of bedwetting has not been successful in establishing continence, parents have generally not reported additional symptoms of instability that might intuitively be expected to accompany failure to achieve a cure (Collins, 1973).

Perhaps the most important implication of the psychodynamic position is that some form of psychotherapy should be applied to the treatment of enuresis, it being held that it is only in this way that the fundamental emotional disorder that is believed to cause the enuresis can be removed. A wide range of theoretical perspectives have been developed within the broad psychodynamic approach, so that there is no single kind of psychotherapy used when treating enuresis. However, various alternative procedures, ranging from verbal counselling and support, to different forms of hypnosis, have in common the assertion that if the enuretic child and/or the child's parents thoroughly explore relevant life experiences under the guidance of a skilled therapist, then they can learn to identify the nature of underlying anxieties and so open the way to overcoming these. It is assumed that, once this has been achieved, then the enuresis will disappear. However, research aimed at evaluating this assertion has not, on the whole, supported it. A number of reviews of the literature available on the efficacy of alternative forms of treatment for bedwetting have reported finding an insufficient number of studies of psychotherapy as a form of treatment which have included adequate samples of enuretics, to permit any firm conclusions regarding this type of treatment (Lovibond, 1964; Kolvin and Taunch, 1973; Baller, 1975). There are, moreover, studies which have found that psychotherapy provides an ineffective method for treating bedwetting. Participants in a study by Werry and Cohrssen (1965) were primary nocturnal enuretic children aged about ten years, with a wetting frequency of at least one wet bed per week. These children were compared with similar enuretic children who were treated later but not at this time, so that they could serve as a control group. One group of 21 children was treated by psychotherapy supplemented by suggestion and encouragement, in six to eight sessions over a period of four months. Twenty-two children in a second experimental group were treated in their own homes using a bedwetting alarm device fitted to the child's bed, as described subsequently in this Chapter when we discuss behavioural theories and methods of treatment associated with these. Treatment in Werry and Cohrssen's study continued until the child had been dry at night for at least one month, or until four months treatment had elapsed. After an initial interview, no further contact was made with the parents or the children in this second group, apart from an occasional telephone call. At the end of four months all parents were contacted by telephone, in order to obtain their records about the frequency of bedwetting during the preceding months for each of the children involved. Results showed that the method of treatment involving the alarm device resulted in a significantly higher rate of improvement (i.e. reduction in the number of bedwetting incidents reported) than was found for either psychotherapy or no-treatment, both of these being ineffective in arresting incontinence.

A similar outcome was subsequently reported by De Leon and Mandell (1966), using a research design very like that in the Werry and Cohrssen study. Once again, three groups of subjects were involved, each receiving either no treatment, psychotherapy, or treatment based on a bedwetting alarm apparatus. At the end of the 90-day experimental period, psychotherapy was found to be as ineffective in eliminating bedwetting as no treatment at all, whereas the alarm device had resulted in a significantly higher success rate. As De Leon and Mandell (1966) were careful to point out, there were many parameters not explored, such as the form of the therapy, the number of therapeutic sessions required for success, the interval between sessions, and individual differences among therapists as to skills and experience. However, these two studies were widely accepted as suggesting that a psychotherapeutic approach does not by itself result in the effective treatment of bedwetting, whereas alternative procedures employing direct behavioural intervention can be markedly more successful. This remains our position and we are not aware of any research in the past 20 years or so since De Leon and Mandell published their work that has produced strong evidence in support of psychodynamic methods of treatment.

In summary, then, bedwetting may sometimes be associated with emotional or behavioural disturbance. However, while it may be useful in some cases to attempt to alleviate emotional or behavioural problems before proceeding with the treatment of bedwetting, it should be emphasized that, in general terms, the nature of an association between such disturbances and bedwetting is by no means clear. In particular, the occurrence of bedwetting should not be seen as necessarily providing evidence for the presence of some underlying conflict, and the great majority of enuretic children do not appear to suffer from any extraordinary degree of emotional or behavioural disorder.

PHYSIOLOGICAL THEORIES AND TREATMENT

Several theories have attempted to account for nocturnal enuresis in terms of a failure to develop physiological control of micturition. Such failure is usually held to be related to either

1. immaturity of the central nervous system (CNS) connections governing bladder control;
2. immaturity of the bladder, resulting in a reduced functional capacity to retain fluid without reflex voiding;
3. profoundly deep sleep or faulty sleep-arousal mechanisms.

Immaturity of the central nervous system (CNS)

The theory that enuresis results from immaturity of neurophysiological structures responsible for bladder control, and that age is the best cure for enuresis, has long-standing and widespread support. As already noted above, epidemiological surveys of three-year-olds have generally found some degree of incontinence among as many as half of all such children, but with a strong general trend towards the reduction of bedwetting with increasing age. Such evidence therefore tends to support the widely followed practice of not intervening with treatment for nocturnal enuresis much before the age of five years, when prevalence has decreased to about 10–15%. It should be pointed out, however, that, even if there is a relatively optimal period for the emergence of dryness during infancy, any interference with this process does appear to have long-term arresting effects. The epidemiological evidence confirms that, among habitual bedwetters beyond about five years of age, the probability of becoming continent without the assistance of therapeutic intervention decreases rapidly.

None the less, there is evidence for the relative physical immaturity of some bedwetters, especially primary enuretic children under the age of five years, when compared with nonenuretic children. Thus, enuretic children have been reported to have slower physical growth on average, higher rates of motor and speech abnormalities and, among older boys, delayed development of secondary sex characteristics.

An increased risk of bedwetting has also been noted among children showing delayed intellectual development or lower than average IQ; and among children with low birthweight, although some research workers have cautioned against accepting low birthweight as evidence for developmental delay. Compared with the norms for the appropriate age group, electroencephalogram (EEG) records of persistent enuretics have also been found to contain diffuse abnormalities, which have sometimes been interpreted as indicating some immaturity of cortical development. It is arguable, however, that the significance of statistically unusual features in the EEGs of children are insufficiently understood to this time, to support the notion of immaturity of cortical development. If it is the case that dysrythmia in the EEG record does reflect immaturity in cortical development, then it should be possible to demonstrate that, among enuretic children with dysrhythmic EEGs, recordings become normal during that time coincident with the spontaneous establishment of bladder control. To this time, however, no adequate test of this prediction has been made.

Evidence for the influence of genetic factors and gender differences on the incidence of enuresis is at least consistent with the view that the development of urinary continence is largely a question of adequate maturation. We have noted in the introductory section to this chapter that a greater prevalence of bedwetting among males than females has been found across a wide range of ages up to about eleven years of age in virtually all epidemiological surveys, with a much more rapid decline in incontinence evident among girls. Furthermore, a higher incidence of childhood enuresis has been found among the parents, siblings and other near relatives of bedwetters, the frequency of occurrence of bedwetting in other members of the family appearing to be related directly to the closeness of the genetic relationship. Bakwin (1971), for example, found concordance for enuresis between identical twins to be double that for fraternal twins. Others have reported that enuretic children are emotionally immature compared with nonenuretic children and this has sometimes been interpreted as evidence for maturational delay.

However, as already pointed out in our discussion of psychodynamic theory, the evidence for such emotional immaturity is problematic and at least the majority of enuretic children seem little different from nonenuretic children in terms of emotional and social adjustment. There is also other evidence contrary to the theory that enuresis is necessarily closely associated with physical immaturity. For example, Oppel et al., (1968), found no relationship between a delay in the development of urinary continence and other developmental milestones. Further, it has frequently been remarked that the development of sphincter control is often intermittent, with periods of relatively good control interspersed with occasional poor control. This pattern is therefore different from the usual pattern of acquiring competence in other developmental disorders. This, together with the contradictory evidence noted above, has led Shaffer (1980) to conclude that the available evidence does not suggest a clear relationship between delays in acquiring urinary continence and other forms of somatic immaturity. MacKeith et al. (1973) have reached much the same conclusion, emphasizing that beyond five years of age immaturity is unlikely to be responsible for continued bedwetting in other than a small number of cases.

Thus, although it does seem likely that delayed maturation is an important factor in the nocturnal incontinence of some younger children, it is important to appreciate that slower maturation does not appear to provide a sufficient explanation for all cases. For example, some children who do not initially progress from incontinence during infancy to consistent dryness in childhood do, none the less, have occasional dry nights and even sustained dry periods across several successive nights. Arguably, the more successive dry nights achieved, the more probably it is that appropriate maturation of the CNS mechanisms responsible for the control of micturition has already occurred. For example, among five-year-old children who have not yet achieved complete nocturnal bladder control, about one third can experience periods of dryness at night lasting from three to nine months. Other evidence that is not consistent with the view that late maturation is predominantly responsible for enuresis is that changing an enuretic child's environment can result in him/her achieving temporary control over bedwetting. Some research has found, for example, that students at boarding school were frequently dry on nights spent in the sick bay, but that they reverted to regular bedwetting when they returned to their usual dormitories. Furthermore, the high rate of rapid success achieved with treatment employing a bedwetting alarm device among nocturnally enuretic children aged seven years or more strongly suggests that, in the majority of such children, maturation of CNS mechanisms has already occurred.

Immaturity of the bladder

Some studies of enuresis have included direct measures of the functional bladder capacity of the children involved to store urine for substantial periods of time without voiding; that is, measurement has been concerned with the quantity of urine retained for a specified duration, rather than with the actual structural size of the bladder. Such measurements are usually achieved by asking parents to collect and to measure the quantity of urine passed on several occasions throughout the course of a week or more. These measures are then averaged, the mean outcome providing the estimate of functional bladder capacity. Evidence from these studies has suggested that, on average, enuretic children have smaller functional bladder capacities than nonenuretic children of the same age, thus providing considerable support for the suggestion that nocturnal enuresis is the result of under-developed functional bladder capacity. The underlying mechanisms for this are not fully understood but it is assumed that, because of the child's developmental delay, the quantity of fluid retained is too small to function as an adequate stimulus for the development of a response inhibiting micturition. Without inhibition of micturition, frequent voidings are necessary, in response to only small volumes of urine accumulating in the bladder.

However, while there appears to be substantial evidence supporting an association between lower functional bladder capacity and enuresis, the nature of this relationship is by no means clear. It is difficult to determine what degree of bladder capacity is adequate for the night-time control of micturition. Frequency of urination during the day does provide an index of day-time functional bladder capacity but it is not a reliable index of a child's night-time capacity to exercise control over the bladder. Obviously, a child who passes urine frequently during the day can nevertheless be dry at night. Furthermore, training procedures designed to distend the bladder, thereby increasing functional bladder capacity, by what is known as 'retention control training', have only been partially successful as a means of eradicating bedwetting. Whereas some researchers have reported that decreased bedwetting has accompanied retention control training, the method has also sometimes resulted in some improvement to functional day-time bladder capacity, but without a significant reduction in bedwetting. The utility of retention control training as a method to accompany other forms of treatment will be discussed in section 2.4. The point to note here is that the relative importance of bladder maturity to the development of nocturnal continence is uncertain; while an underdeveloped functional bladder capacity may be involved in many cases of bedwetting, it is unlikely that this provides a sufficient explanation for all cases. Thus, frequency distributions of measured functional bladder capacity among enuretic and nonenuretic children do overlap to a considerable extent. Moreover, especially when older enuretic children are considered, it seems more plausible that other factors will also be involved.

Depth of sleep
The belief that bedwetting is a consequence of the child's tendency to sleep deeply and be difficult to wake is very common among the parents of enuretic children, and there is a good deal of anecdotal evidence to this effect. Despite such indications, however, clinical observations of the relationship between depth of sleep and bedwetting have not resulted in clear support for this idea. Thus, comparisons between enuretic and nonenuretic children for ease of arousability from sleep, using an auditory stimulus like a buzzer or calling

the child's name to awaken the child, have produced contradictory results. Some studies have found that enuretic children take longer to awaken than nonenuretic controls but others have found that the waking time in the two groups is essentially the same. We have recently investigated the deep sleep hypothesis, comparing arousability among enuretic nine to ten-year-olds and nonenuretic siblings or first cousins.* The alarm which we developed for this purpose is connected in the usual way to a commercially available moisture-sensitive rubber pad. The small battery-operated alarm unit has been modified to include an alarm clock. The clock was preset to sound the alarm at one, four and seven hours after sleep onset on different nights. Enuretic children were additionally awakened by each wetting accident since this also sounded the alarm. A stopwatch was activated when the alarm began to sound, so that the time for it to be switched off by the child was measured precisely. This duration was taken as the index of arousability. In one condition the alarm was a loud buzzer and in an alternative condition it was a prerecording of the mother's voice calling the child by name and urging him or her to wake up.

We found that enuretic children were significantly slower to arouse than the nonenuretic controls, suggesting that, in general terms, enuretic children do sleep more deeply than comparable nonenuretic children. Whether the auditory signal was an alarm or a recording of the mother's voice made no difference to the outcome. A detailed analysis of arousability during wet and dry nights, however, found no evidence to link wet incidents with periods of deepest sleep, the enuretic children taking on average about the same time to awaken to the alarm following an accident as when aroused by a prescheduled alarm, not associated with bedwetting. Moreover, notable features of the data were, first, very wide differences between individuals in waking time, with light and heavy sleepers in both groups; secondly,

* The data in this study were collected by Ms L. Chamberlain and formed the basis of her Honours research thesis in the Department of Psychology, University of Adelaide, during 1986.

within-individual differences were also very wide, the deepest sleepers none the less waking quickly on some occasions.

Most empirical data relating to sleep and enuresis have been obtained in studies employing electroencephalographic (EEG) recordings of electrical activity in the brain during sleep. The major issues of interest in relation to bedwetting have been, firstly, whether the overall patterns of EEG activity during the sleep of enuretic and nonenuretic children differ in fundamental ways and, secondly, whether bedwetting episodes occur predominantly during stages corresponding to deeper sleep. To this time, such studies have not generally revealed reliable differences between the sleep patterns of enuretic and nonenuretic children, both groups spending about the same time in various stages of sleep identified as reflecting relative depth of sleep. One recent study has even reported that enuretic boys spent significantly more time in relatively shallow sleep than nonenuretic controls; a finding which is of course the opposite to what is predicted by the deep sleep hypothesis.

The evidence in respect of the second issue does not support the idea that bedwetting is confined to times of deepest sleep. Although enuretic episodes have been found to be more commonly associated with deeper stages, and bedwetting incidents are rare during the stage associated with lightest sleep (the rapid-eye-movement, or REM, stage), several studies have observed that bedwetting does occur during all other stages of sleep. Furthermore, at least one study has found that patterns of sleep among enuretic boys were not linked in any way to bedwetting incidents, remaining essentially the same whether the children wet the bed or remained dry.

According to Broughton (1968), the essential prediction is not that bedwetting should be associated with a particular stage of deep sleep, but rather that bedwetting should accompany the transition from deepest sleep to lighter stages. His suggestion was that bedwetting is better regarded as a consequence of a failure to arouse from sleep in time to control micturition and several researchers have made observations consistent with this idea. Thus, studies have confirmed that bedwetting occurs during arousal from deep sleep and that enuretic children are harder to arouse than appropriate non-enuretic controls. There is evidence that, in addition to being unresponsive to external stimulation, enuretic children can also be relatively unresponsive to introceptive stimulation from a distended and rapidly contracting bladder. De Perri and Meduri (1972) made simultaneous recordings of brain (EEG) and bladder activity among bedwetters and non-bedwetters with full bladders, during both spontaneous and pharmacologically induced sleep. Reflex micturition occurred without clinical signs of wakefulness in the enuretic group but with transient EEG evidence of arousal. Non-bedwetters on the other hand woke without accident, their records showing definite electro-clinical arousal for bladder pressures below threshold levels of reflex voiding. Thus, the weight of evidence is consistent with Broughton's suggestion, that the sleep-arousal system of bedwetters is in some way significantly less effective than it is among children developing normal control. If so, then it may be that effective forms of treatment, like those employing the bed-pad and alarm device to be described in the account of behavioural theories and treatment below, derive some part of their success from their capacity to improve the arousability of the child.

Medical treatment
Medical practitioners most commonly prescribe either of two treatments for bedwetting, the choice being determined by the child's age. If it is assumed that the bedwetting is the consequence of immaturely developed physiological mechanisms governing bladder control, no formal treatment may be recommended for younger children, other than the advice that the child will eventually outgrow the problem. However, although surveys of prevalence do suggest that some children with established enuresis will spontaneously cease to wet the bed as they grow older, at present one cannot predict at what age an enuretic child will become dry spontaneously; nor is it possible to identify the 2% who will continue to wet the bed into their latter teenage years and beyond.

Another frequently practised method of treatment, especially with older enuretic children, is to prescribe some form of medication. Only one review (Johnson, 1980) of this form of treatment has appeared since the earlier very comprehensive review by Blackwell and Currah (1973). These reviews were in substantial agreement, with results for a wide range of prescribed drugs suggesting that most forms of medication have not been found to be effective in controlling bedwetting. Only the tricyclic antidepressants have been consistently found to be better than placebo, the most commonly used and extensively studied medication being imipramine (Tofranil). Such drugs possibly work by increasing arousability from sleep in response to stimulation from a filling bladder, and may also act at the level of the bladder and sphincter, relaxing the detrusor muscle and thereby increasing bladder capacity and contracting the sphincter. It has also been suggested, in line with psychodynamic theory, that the drug may act to reduce the child's underlying depression, for which bedwetting is regarded as a symptom. However, empirical evidence relevant to these explanations is inconclusive. The capacity of tricyclic antidepressants to change arousability from sleep or to increase bladder capacity has not been reliably demonstrated and, as already discussed at length above, there is little evidence to justify regarding all or even most cases of enuresis as being caused, even in part, by underlying depression.

The drug Tofranil and similar tricyclic antidepressants usually do reduce bedwetting frequency fairly soon, with improvement typically being found during the first week of treatment. However, not infrequently, further improvements are not made, with bedwetting incidents levelling out at perhaps two or three wet nights per week. While a reduction of this order in the number of bedwetting episodes is usually welcomed at first, and is frequently found to be statistically significant in studies making pre-treatment and post-treatment comparisons, it none the less eventually comes to be seen as unsatisfactory by most parents, who inevitably hope that the child will become completely continent. In fact, a complete initial remission is usually obtained for less than

50% of those cases treated by medication and, at follow-up (for example after six months) sustained continence is typically achieved by as few as 10–20% of these cases. Frequently, too, relapse tends to occur immediately following the withdrawal of medication, an obvious shortcoming of this kind of treatment.

A further shortcoming of drug therapy is the possibility of imipramine poisoning, not only for the enuretic child but also among siblings having access to tablets. In the short-term, side effects like reduced concentration, restlessness and increased irritability have frequently been reported. The longer-term effects of such drugs are as yet not known, and are therefore obviously of concern.

In summary, the mechanism by which tricyclic antidepressants influence enuresis remains unknown. The anticholinergic properties of these drugs may extend the storage capacity of urine in the bladder before voiding, although other possibilities, including antidepressant and arousing effects, have been suggested. However, treatment by drugs, without any additional procedures, produces complete continence in only a minority of cases.

BEHAVIOURAL THEORIES AND TREATMENT

Somewhat like physiological theories, behavioural theories attribute nocturnal enuresis to a failure to develop cortical control over subcortical effector mechanisms. However, instead of involving processes like neural maturation, under-developed functional bladder capacity or faulty arousal from sleep, as already discussed in the previous sections, behavioural theorists emphasize the role of learning in the development of processes necessary for achieving continence. Most psychologists adopting a behavioural theoretical perspective on the treatment of bedwetting prefer to use some version of the bed-pad and alarm method, although this is not always the case. There is now a small number of reports in the literature about the efficacy of hypnosis as the basis for treatment of bedwetting although, on our reading about this topic, it is still too early to determine how effective such treatment is and we have no direct experience with these procedures. The aim when using hypnosis is to use suggestions to aid the child to gain control of a range of behaviours associated with night-time toileting. Butler (1987) has provided a brief account of the application of both hypnotherapy and self-hypnosis. He suggests that there is a better chance of success with older children, although we note that overall success rates do not appear to compare with those commonly achieved with the bedwetting alarm.

Parents, of course, commonly attempt to alleviate their child's bedwetting by the application of a number of behavioural methods readily available to them, like punishment following bedwetting accidents, waking the child at various times throughout the night in an attempt to prevent an accident from occurring, and rewarding dry nights when these do occur. In the great majority of cases, however, these procedures are not effective in producing a cure, although parents sometimes find that they can reduce wetting incidents somewhat for short periods of time. None of these procedures, however, compares favourably with available alarm procedures. For an overview of simple behavioural measures for dealing with bedwetting, the reader is also directed to Smith and Smith (1987). These management procedures include hypnotherapy, anxiety reduction, night-time waking schedules, fluid restriction, star charts and other rewards, punishments and dietary manipulation.

Standard conditioning with a bed-pad and alarm

The processes involved in achieving bladder control are complex and the importance of neural maturation is beyond question but it seems clear that, in addition, learning is involved. Various conceptualizations have been suggested as to the nature of these learning processes which are assumed to supplement neural maturation, but the essential idea is that bedwetting is the consequence of some habit deficiency, either because appropriate learning has not yet developed, or because, somehow, past learning has broken down. Thus, the enuretic child must learn to control reflex voiding, and behavioural treatment procedures aim to arouse appropriate responding under careful prescribed conditions.

According to Lovibond's (1964) influential review of nocturnal enuresis, for the majority of enuretic children the problem is the consequence of the absence of environmental conditions which are necessary for learning the response of sphincter inhibition. In addition, in some cases a child may be particularly resistant to learning, perhaps because of lower intelligence or because of some other aberration associated with the CNS. Lovibond also recognized that a failure to develop control may be due to high anxiety or nervous tension which interfere with efficient learning or which can result in the breakdown of previously established linkages, but he considered that this would be so in only a minority of cases.

Behavioural therapists have analysed environmental conditions associated with learning bladder control in an attempt to advance understanding about the cause of enuresis. Treatment procedures are derived from the theory that achieving continence requires the learning of the discriminative cues that permit the inhibition of urination until appropriate toileting is possible.

Strong support for the view that learning plays an essential role in the attainment of bladder control comes from the well-established high rate of success obtained with the treatment of enuresis by various urine-alarm devices. This procedure relies on an alarm to awaken the enuretic child immediately after urination has occurred.* Thus, the alarm sounds immediately when the first traces of urine close an open circuit built into a moisture-sensitive, specially designed detector mat or pad, on which the child sleeps. The most common kinds of detector involve two electrodes (anode and cathode), either in the form of two mats made of metal mesh,

---

* Mountjoy et al. (1984) include an historical account of anti-enuretic devices patented in the United States. They describe what appears to be the only plan to date for an apparatus designed to predict micturition before it has occurred, by detecting a particular finger flexing response claimed always to precede an enuretic incident.

or a single moulded rubber pad with the metal electrodes embedded within it. This kind of device is variously described in the literature as a 'bell-and-pad', 'urine-alarm', 'buzzer', 'enuresis alarm', 'anti-enuretic device', etc. The form of treatment based on equipment of this kind is commonly referred to as the **standard conditioning** method, and modern versions of this are essentially the same as the first systematic treatment method for nocturnal enuresis, based on conditioning principles, that was described by Mowrer and Mowrer (1938).* They argued that enuresis results from a failure to acquire the habit of responding to a filling bladder in the night by awakening and/or contracting the urethral sphincter muscles to prevent reflexive voiding; the bed-pad with alarm procedure was a logical outcome of their theoretical analysis, although the potential therapeutic effects of an apparatus of this kind had earlier been recognized in 1904 by Pfaundler.

Treatment of nocturnal enuresis by an alarm device involves having the child sleep on a moisture-sensitive detector pad which is placed under the bed sheet and connected to a battery-operated alarm, like a bell, a buzzer, or, under some circumstances, a visual stimulus. Where the alarm system involves two mats, the bottom one is normally laid on a cotton sheet covering a waterproof sheet which protects the mattress. The lower mat is separated from the upper mat by a flannelette draw sheet. The whole arrangement is then covered and tucked in position by a cotton draw sheet, as illustrated in the next Chapter (Figure 2.2, p. 57). Nylon sheeting is best avoided since it can cause perspiration, which can result in false alarms. If wetting during sleep occurs then the alarm rings, sufficiently loudly to awaken the child immediately, so that the child can consciously inhibit further micturition. Modern equipment follows the same basic

* According to Mountjoy *et al.* (1984), the principle of using moisture to conduct electricity, and so close an open circuit, was first applied in the latter part of the nineteenth century to the design of alarm systems capable of detecting burst water pipes in buildings, thereby preventing damage. A USA patent to apply the same principle to the detection of bedwetting was first filed in 1905.

design as that employed by the Mowrers, but now incorporates more recent technological advances which have virtually eliminated a number of problems encountered with earlier versions of the apparatus. Thus, there is now no danger of burning or ulceration to the surface of the skin as a consequence of contact with the electrodes if these are embedded in the pad, and recent recommendations about levels of electric current are followed (Coote, 1965; Greaves, 1969; Neal and Coote, 1969; Pfeiffer and Lloyd, 1978). We have included an account of a number of currently available commercial devices at the end of this Chapter.

Mowrer and Mowrer sought to explain the effectiveness of treatment by the bed-pad and alarm procedure in terms of the reflexive mechanisms formulated more than 60 years ago by the Russian physiologist Ivan Pavlov, as a consequence of his pioneering studies in classical conditioning. The Mowrers reasoned that increasing tension in the detrusor muscle would act as an unconditional stimulus (US_1), to elicit the unconditional response (UR_1) of reflex voiding. They also regarded the alarm, triggered by bedwetting, as an unconditional stimulus (US_2) which would produce two unconditional responses; it would result in the inhibition of urination by eliciting reflexive sphincter contraction (UR_2) but it would also wake the child (UR_3). According to their theory, pairing the two unconditional stimuli would result in increasing detrusor muscle tension acquiring the status of a conditional stimulus (CS). Thus, because it occurred in close contiguity with the alarm, tension in the detrusor muscle would, as a consequence of learning, gradually produce the required conditional responses of inhibiting urination because of sphincter contraction (CR_2) and waking the child (CR_3). Since increasing tension in the detrusor muscle represents a gradient of intensity, the Mowrers reasoned that, as treatment progressed, the reflex act of voiding would become increasingly inhibited by less powerful signals of detrusor muscle tension, until the child would wake without having urinated, before the alarm was triggered. In this way, as the CS became established by the conditioning procedure, the child would achieve complete continence during sleep.

The adequacy of an explanation in terms of classical conditioning has been in serious doubt since Lovibond's authorative examination of this issue more than 20 years ago (Lovibond, 1964). As Lovibond made clear, unlike the CS in the classical Pavlovian model, tension in the detrusor muscle of the bladder is not originally neutral with respect to micturition but, in fact, is a US for reflexive voiding. The Mowrers' theoretical account did not explain how detrusor tension acquired the status of a CS – or why the alarm did not. Furthermore, as Pavlov's experiments in conditioning demonstrated, a CS does not retain the capacity to elicit the CR unless it is periodically paired with the US. If this is not done, experimental extinction occurs. Thus, according to the classical conditioning model, dryness following initial treatment would not be sustained indefinitely. Certainly, it is the case that relapses following initially successful treatment has always been an important problem-feature of the bed-pad and alarm procedure. However, it is also clearly the case that a majority of children treated in this way do achieve permanent continence following initial treatment.

A third problem for this model raised by Lovibond was that some children respond to conditioning without ever waking to urinate. Such cases are rare but that any occur is something that the Mowrers' theory of classical conditioning cannot account for since waking to urinate is an integral part of the conditioned response formed to bladder distension (CS). Furthermore, the Mowrers' explanation could not account for the fact that children eventually sleep through the night without waking or wetting.

As we shall see when discussing the Dry-Bed Training procedures (pp. 34–40) these considerations were not merely of academic interest and they were, in fact, to stimulate a lot of research during the next two decades that would help to improve the reliability of treatment methods. Lovibond's explanation for the effectiveness of treatment utilizing the bed-pad with alarm procedure was based on a form of operant conditioning theory, which emphasizes the role of the consequences that follow specific behaviours in either strengthening or decreasing the probability of the future occurrence of those behaviours. In particular, he proposed that the treatment of bedwetting by the alarm device is properly described in terms of passive avoidance learning, rather than as classical conditioning. The essential part of Lovibond's argument was that the state of being woken in response to an alarm is essentially unpleasant, and that the bed-pad with alarm procedure successfully links this wakening response to the alarm. Eventually, so as to avoid the aversive consequences of the alarm, the child learns to contract the sphincter and, if necessary, to wake without wetting. The act of waking, however, is not essential to the learning process, so that Lovibond's explanation could cope with those small numbers of children who respond to treatment without waking to urinate. All that the avoidance theory assumes is that waking to an alarm is aversive for those children, as for others – a plausible assumption since it is virtually inconceivable that all children would not, at some time, have experienced a sudden awakening from sleep. On the basis of research aimed at describing passive avoidance learning, Lovibond argued that this conditioning avoidance response should be very resistant to extinction. In other words, once learning has occurred it could be maintained, even indefinitely, without further exposure to the alarm.

Several reviews of research done since the publication of Lovibond's book have confirmed that the bed-pad and alarm procedure is very effective in arresting nocturnal enuresis (Johnson, 1980; Butler, 1987). Bedwetting is arrested in about 75–80% of cases treated in this way, with the duration of treatment in most instances ranging from about five to twelve weeks. Methods based on the alarm device have been consistently found to arrest bedwetting more effectively than training which attempts to improve control over micturition by increasing the capacity of the bladder without voiding, or by the application of drug therapies, or a wide range of psychotherapeutic approaches aiming to provide supportive counselling.

This success notwithstanding, it remains the case that perhaps as many as 20% of children treated by an alarm procedure fail to achieve permanent continence within a reasonable treatment period, and there are certainly still some practical problems associated with the standard bed-pad and alarm procedure. It can be inconvenient and frustrating for parents and child alike, particularly when the child wets several times in the night or if false alarms occur because of excessive sweating or machine malfunction. Although rechargable appliances are sometimes available, most alarm units in use today are powered by low-voltage, dry-cell batteries and if these are allowed to run low the unit can fail to function, thereby effectively disrupting treatment. Treatment can also be sabotaged if the child switches off the alarm before going to sleep, or if the parents or the child forget to switch it on. Some children fail to awaken to the alarm, at least initially, and special arrangements may be required in order to overcome this. (A possible solution in such cases is to set the alarm with an extension to the parents' room so that it wakes a parent, who then wakes the child. If this is done, then the alarm is best left ringing by the parents, so that the child must get out of bed and switch it off – at the extension in the child's room. This last point is important; the parents should always leave it to the child to switch off the alarm, assuming that the child is mature enough to do this responsibly. Usually, this arrangement is not required beyond the first few nights, however, after which most children begin to respond to the alarm.) A single wetting incident after several successive dry nights can be extremely disappointing to the child and to the parents, and they may become discouraged about persevering with treatment when this occurs. In Chapter 3 we have outlined a number of cases where these kind of problems have been encountered, together with brief accounts of how we have attempted to deal with them. In fact, it now seems clear that reasons like those summarized here will result in failure to persist with treatment in about a third of all cases entering treatment programmes, unless treatment is supported by close supervision from a clinician.

The influence of many different subject variables on response to treatment involving the alarm device has been thoroughly investigated but few such variables have been found to influence outcome to a significant, reliable extent. Thus, the effectiveness of this procedure does not generally appear to depend on the frequency of prior bedwetting, the sex of the child, or on whether the enuresis was primary or secondary in form. Nor does there seem to be any reliable difference between the responses to this form of treatment of children known to be suffering from emotional disturbances, when compared with non-disturbed enuretic children, at least with regards to the percentage cured or the speed with which an initial arrest is achieved. However, some results from comparisons of this kind have suggested that disturbed children show a greater likelihood of relapse following a period of continence. Less favourable outcomes have also been associated with high levels of maternal anxiety and disturbed family backgrounds and with unsatisfactory housing conditions.

The most important shortcoming of treatment employing the bed-pad and alarm procedure remains the substantial number of children who do resume wetting the bed, after having achieved continence for a significant period of time like two or three weeks. A wide range of rates for relapse following standard conditioning have been reported, ranging from about 15% to 70%, but an average relapse rate from the many studies now available from the considerable literature on this topic is approximately 40%.

There are some indications that relapse is more probable among cases where day-time urinary problems exist, or where individual emotional or behavioural problems or the presence of marital discord or other family difficulties can be identified. Some studies, too, have suggested that a higher frequency of bedwetting before treatment commences will increase the likelihood of subsequent relapse. However, at this stage any conclusions about this issue are, at most, speculative. It seems quite clear that the age and sex of the child and the general pattern of bedwetting are not associated with the probability of relapse but it remains the case that attempts to develop reliable predictors for relapse following conditioning treatment have not yet been successful.

One of two procedures, both adjunctive to the bed-pad

with alarm method, has generally been followed as a countermeasure to the problem of relapse. One involves employing the alarm so that, instead of the alarm ringing for each wetting incident, it sounds for only some, following some variable proportion of wets. This is termed an 'intermittent schedule'. The theoretical rationale for this approach derives from basic principles of learning which have established that a response that has been reinforced only intermittently is much more resistant to extinction. According to this theory, the response in question is the appropriate inhibition of micturition and the form of reinforcement is the successful avoidance of the aversive alarm. Learning achieved by partial reinforcement should therefore be very resistant to extinction – that is, to relapse. The second procedure often employed in combination with standard conditioning is called 'overlearning training', which involves increasing the child's fluid intake, with the aim of improving bladder retention capacity as the conditioning treatment proceeds. Both of these procedures have been found to be effective in reducing the number of relapses following treatment with the bed-pad and alarm device, with overlearning training being somewhat superior to intermittent reinforcement. However, both alternatives have been found to significantly increase the time required to attain dryness in the first place – by at least 25% and perhaps even by as much as 65% in some instances. This is obviously a major problem for all involved, child, parents and therapists alike. Faced with the prospect of an extension to treatment of something like three to seven weeks, it is not surprising that some families opt for the bed-pad and alarm method, without the inclusion of additional procedures, hoping that for their child relapse will not prove to be a problem. None the less, relapse does remain a problem with the standard conditioning procedure.

Dry-Bed Training

The Dry-Bed Training procedure was first developed by researchers working with Professor N.H. Azrin at Illinois (e.g. Azrin, *et al.*, 1974). This approach views the development of nocturnal continence as an operant learning process in which particular social and motivational factors serve as rewards which will increase the probability that appropriate control of micturition will occur. Within this theoretical framework, therefore, social and motivational considerations are regarded as being as important as sensitivity to bladder sensation; and enuresis is held to result from insufficient social reinforcement and inhibitory influences. In line with this theory, Azrin and his coworkers have incorporated a number of operant training procedures which emphasize positive reinforcement for nocturnal bladder control as well as aversive consequences immediately following bedwetting episodes, into one comprehensive programme for treatment. The urine-alarm apparatus forms part of the procedure followed but is regarded essentially as a convenient means for reliably identifying that a bedwetting event has occurred, so that appropriate punishment can be applied immediately, rather than as a method for providing direct conditioning of the bladder sphincter. Punishment within this programme consists of four separate elements; first, being awakened by the alarm; secondly, verbal admonishment following a bedwetting episode; thirdly, a demanding cleanliness training procedure, which requires that the child changes wet sheets, deposits them in the laundry and completely re-makes the bed before returning to sleep; and, fourthly, an extremely demanding positive practice routine whereby the child must first count to 50 and then go to the toilet, this practice being repeated 20 times once cleanliness training has been per-formed. However, Dry-Bed Training also emphasizes the importance of a range of positive reinforcements which are contingent upon nocturnal control, such special rewards being given by the parents immediately the child wakes after a dry night. In addition to reinforcement and punishment procedures, Dry-Bed Training includes a number of addi-tional features derived from other forms of treatment. These are regular night-time awakenings, increased fluid intake before bedtime together with practice in retaining urine before voiding, and practice in correct night-time toileting behav-iour. An initial intensive training session which takes all night is done during the first night of treatment by a professional trainer who sleeps in the child's home on this occasion. The parents then take over the supervision of the programme for subsequent nights, until the child becomes continent. The Dry-Bed Training programme therefore represents a very eclectic approach to the problem of bedwetting which, although based essentially on operant conditioning theory, also incorporates a variety of treatment procedures which have been adopted from a range of theories.

In recent years a good deal of research has sought to evaluate Dry-Bed Training, comparing this approach which, in effect, includes the bed-pad and alarm procedure within a wide-based eclectic programme, with the standard conditioning method – the bed-pad and alarm without including these additional features. This research has generally found that Dry-Bed Training is more effective than standard conditioning, arresting bedwetting in less time. However, the extent to which treatment time is reduced is almost certainly not as marked as was initially thought, with most more recent researchers reporting success rates that are less remarkable than was first reported by the Azrin group. Another very important concern of this research, which we have focused on in our own work, has been the relevance of the bed-pad and alarm apparatus within Dry-Bed Training. Although Azrin has concluded that incorporating this device does not make an essential contribution to the success of Dry-Bed Training, we have since established that this is not so, demonstrating effectively that children undergoing a modified Dry-Bed Training programme that does not include any alarm procedure do not, except in rare instances, achieve complete dryness. Such children may, on average, show a substantial drop in the frequency of bedwetting during early training, but thereafter there is no further improvement. Most such children maintain a plateau of reduced bedwetting but continue to wet the bed regularly and only a very few become completely dry.

We have also investigated the effectiveness of the standard conditioning method with the full Dry-Bed Training procedure including the urine-alarm, and administered by a professional trainer who stays overnight in the child's home during the first night (the procedure recommended by Azrin); or by a professional trainer with the child in hospital for the first night and following the full procedure which includes an alarm; or by the child's parents at home taking full responsibility for the initial night of intensive training and under conditions which either included or excluded an alarm. We have found Dry-Bed Training with an alarm included to be equally effective under all conditions but have found it to be only marginally more effective than the standard conditioning procedure involving just the bed-pad and alarm with regular telephone contact between the child's family and the therapist, in terms of both the proportion of children successfully treated and the overall speed of treatment. Moreover, although Dry-Bed Training without an alarm resulted in significantly fewer bedwettings than in the control group not given any treatment, this modified procedure was much less effective than any of the alarm-based treatments.

In spite of the impressive results obtained for Dry-Bed Training, in terms of both the proportion of cases who achieve initial arrest of bedwetting and the speed with which most children achieve complete arrest, this procedure does pose a number of problems for large-scale use in clinical practice that do not apply to the same degree in the case of the standard conditioning method. The major difficulty is that the Dry-Bed Training programme is very time-consuming to follow because it involves a complicated schedule of tasks that can confuse some children and their parents and therefore undermine their motivation to persist with treatment. Furthermore, although we have successfully demonstrated that parents can be used instead of a professional trainer in the home during the initial all-night session without reducing the programme's effectiveness, the fact remains that training parents to do this properly is very time-consuming. In our experience, instructing parents to take full responsibility for Dry-Bed Training requires at least 60–90 minutes, compared with the 20–30 minutes usually required in order to instruct the parents and the child in the standard conditioning procedure.

We have attempted to address this limitation, by instructing the parents of enuretic children to administer Dry-Bed Training within small group settings. Results from these training programmes have been very satisfactory. None the less, even with the advantages of small group instruction, Dry-Bed Training still places heavy demands on parents and children, especially during the initial phase of training. Considerable effort is necessary to persuade children to comply with instructions, especially during the positive practice components which, because of their repetitive, time-consuming nature, generally come to be quickly regarded by both children and their parents as particularly aversive. For these reasons, we have attempted to delineate which aspects of Dry-Bed Training, in addition to the alarm, contribute most to its overall effectiveness, with the intention of subsequently simplifying the procedure. Our research on this matter has suggested that the effects of the three main components, identified as the waking schedule, retention control training, and positive practice, are cumulative, so that the more components added to the alarm-only procedure, the better the therapeutic response. None the less, from a perspective of practical, significant gain, retention control training and positive practice can be eliminated from the Dry-Bed Training schedule without sacrificing its overall effectiveness to any significant degree. Gains from these two components are only marginal and the combination of the waking schedule together with the urine-alarm is virtually as effective as the complete Dry-Bed Training programme. To summarize the outcome of this research then, the bed-pad and alarm supported by the waking schedule is more effective than the bed-pad and alarm alone but difference in length of treatment necessary is not great in most cases.

For the purpose of practical application, these findings are the most important. They mean that the heavy demands of the full Dry-Bed Training programme can be reduced substantially, without noticeably sacrificing the programme's effectiveness. Although including the waking schedule does require more of the child than the standard conditioning method, additional demands are only substantial on the initial night, during which the child is awakened hourly for toileting. However, following this initial intensive all-night session, on subsequent nights the child is only awakened once during the night and most parents and children appear to cope satisfactorily with this requirement. Indeed, in our experience, many parents report that, prior to bringing a child for treatment, they have previously employed the practice of regularly waking the child during the night, in an attempt to manage the child's bedwetting. On the other hand, if the parents or child prefer not to follow the waking schedule then, in most cases, this is not likely to prolong treatment by more than a week or two.

Adequate data on relapse following Dry-Bed Training are as yet very limited but, on the basis of our own research, it would appear to be the case that, like standard conditioning, Dry-Bed Training is associated with a high relapse rate. Our findings about the use of Dry-Bed Training without the inclusion of an alarm differ substantially from reports by Azrin and his colleagues. They have claimed that bedwetting can be eliminated effectively by a training programme similar to the original Dry-Bed Training schedule but without including any procedure involving an alarm and with some modifications to the intensive training session and the way parents were instructed. However, our research into this matter has found no evidence to support this assertion. On the contrary, we have found that, although the occasional child does achieve dryness when treated in this way, and the overall incidence of bedwetting is somewhat reduced, most cases do not achieve complete arrest, even for a short time. One possible explanation for this difference is that Azrin's subjects have generally been much younger than the children treated by us, and therefore more likely to have been more responsive to most forms of therapy. The issue should not be regarded as settled yet and, clearly, further research is required. At present, however, our view remains that the most effective forms of treatment for bedwetting utilize a bed-pad and alarm but, at the same time, it seems clear that a number of operant variables are effective in reducing bedwetting. Thus, a simple theoretical explanation in terms of either classical or instrumental (i.e. operant) conditioning is not sufficient. Forms of social intervention, like training in rapid awakening, practice in withholding urination, massed practice in correct night-time toileting behaviour, and differential social reinforcement for wet or dry nights, can contribute to the overall effectiveness of treatment, in addition to the specific effects of the urine-alarm. Moreover, as emphasized by Butler (1987), the perspectives which the child and the parents hold about bedwetting and the treatment programme will also be important determinants of treatment outcome. Treatment is unlikely to succeed unless the child actively wishes to achieve dryness, or if the child is actually resistant to change – as occasionally seems to be the case in those rare instances where the child apparently continues wetting deliberately. If a parent (particularly the mother) displays intolerance towards the demands of the treatment programme, or about the slow progress of the child, then early withdrawal from treatment is likely to follow unless the therapist can move to reduce dissatisfaction. A major shortcoming of current large-scale bedwetting clinics is that as many as 30% of families entering a treatment programme discontinue prematurely.

Summary of conditioning treatments
There is now substantial evidence that conditioning treatments of enuresis based on the bed-pad and alarm device are superior to psychotherapy and medication. However, alternative conditioning models are available and, when deciding whether to provide, for example, Dry-Bed Training, standard conditioning, or some other combination of training procedures, the therapist is faced with considerations about the speed and endurance of treatment and the comparative ease with which each of these methods could be implemented. Taking these matters into account, we have concluded that standard conditioning based on the bed-pad and alarm, with regular back-up by a therapist, and possibly combined with a night-time waking schedule, provides the most cost-effective treatment for large-scale clinical practice. A more detailed protocol for the management of bedwetting in this way is set out in section 2.4. At the present time,

however, it must be acknowledged that for reasons which are not yet understood, as many as one in five children treated in this way will not respond satisfactorily to treatment.

CURRENT COMMERCIAL BEDWETTING DEVICES

Within Australia, the United Kingdom and the USA, the three countries surveyed here, many different brands of urine-alarm systems are currently available. However, there are surprisingly few published studies that have evaluated and compared the effectiveness of the available equipment, or even provided details of where such equipment can be purchased. We have surveyed the literature up to this time, with the aim of providing guidance to a potential purchaser of commercially available bedwetting equipment. The list of alarm systems reviewed here is certainly not exhaustive but it does cover a broad spectrum of types of alarm. Furthermore, while the country of origin of the equipment reviewed is either the UK, the USA or Australia, most of these systems are now available world-wide. With the exception of the Ramsey–Coote system, we have not included details about the cost of equipment since all prices published in these sources are now at least four years out of date.

An unpublished report entitled *Nocturnal Enuresis: Management, Systems and Equipment Evaluation* has been produced by the Oxford Regional Health Authority in the UK.* This provides information about the management of bedwetting, obtained from 174 Health Authorities throughout the UK, most of the report being devoted to the description and evaluation of various bed-pad and alarm systems, though no attempt is made to identify a 'best buy'. Twenty-six different alarm systems are identified, with detailed comments and comparison results from tests during 1982 for twelve of them. Accessories to standard alarm systems, such as attachments to increase auditory stimulation, relay alarms

---

* This report by Hunt *et al.* can be obtained for a fee by writing to Enuresis Research, 54 Armour Hill, Tilehurst, Reading, Berks, RG3 6JH.

Table 1.1 Enuresis alarm equipment available in the UK.

Alarm model	Manufacturer's address
1. Astric Dry-Bed	Astric Products Ltd., Astric House, 148 Lewes Road, Brighton, Sussex BN2 3LG.
2. Connevan's Alarm	Connevan's Ltd., 1–3 Norbury Road, Reigate, Surrey RH2 96Y.
3. Chiron Mark III	Down's Surgical Co. Ltd., Church Path, Mitcham, Surrey CR4 3UE.
4. Down's Mark V	Down's Surgical Co. Ltd., Church Path, Mitcham, Surrey CR4 3UE.
5. Eastleigh A1P	N.H. Eastwood & Son Ltd., 70 Nursery Road, Southgate, London, NH14 5QH.
6. Eastleigh Ministry of Health (MOH) 1P	N.H. Eastwood & Son Ltd., 70 Nursery Road, Southgate, London, NH14 5QH.
7. Eastleigh Dri-Nite	N.H. Eastwood & Son Ltd., 70 Nursery Road, Southgate, London, NH14 5QH.
8. Eastleigh SM1	N.H. Eastwood & Son Ltd., 70 Nursery Road, Southgate, London, NH14 5QH.
9. Headingley alternating pulse alarm with test button	Headingley Scientific Sciences, 20 Cottage Road, Leeds LS6 4DD.[a]
10. Urilarm – hospital and deluxe models	F. Gulliver (Devices) Ltd., The Mews, 49/51 Station Road, London.[a]
11. Malem electronic bedwetting alarm and toilet trainer	Malem Medical, 4 Rufford Road, Sherwood, Nottingham NG5 2NR. (Distributed by Nottingham Medical Aids Ltd., 17 Ludlow Hill Road, Melton Road, West Bridgford, Nottingham NG2 6HD).
12. Wessex with test button and accessories	Wessex Medical Equipment Co. Ltd., Alma Road, Romsey, Hampshire.[a]

[a] This is the later 1983 address published in Goel *et al.* (1984).

to other rooms and alternative stimulation (e.g. the use of vibrators) are also discussed. Manufacturers and their addresses are provided. The twelve systems are as set out in Table 1.1.

The authors of the Oxford Regional Health Authority report issue a warning that the mat current obtained with three of the alarms in Table 1.1 was outside recommended specifications. These were the Eastleigh A1P, Eastleigh Dri-Nite and the Urilarm hospital and deluxe models. In addition, the authors consider that because the Malem device is essentially a small sensor, worn within a cotton nappy pad, it may be better suited to the treatment of diurnal enuresis or to toilet training than to the treatment of nocturnal enuresis.

A second recent review of commercially available enuresis alarms in the UK has been produced by Goel *et al.* (1984). In this study, 100 nocturnally enuretic children were treated under supervised trial conditions with nine commonly used enuresis alarm systems: the Astric Dry-Bed Mark II; Chiron Mark III; Eastleigh Ministry of Health (MOH) I; Eastleigh MOH I and Booster; Headingley; Headingley with Silent Wakener; Headingley with extension; Urilarm deluxe; and Wessex. The method of allocating the children participating in this study to a particular alarm group is not described in the article, and the numbers in each group varied from five children who used the Headingley alarm with extension to fourteen children who used the Astric Dry-Bed Mark II apparatus.

These nine alarm systems were evaluated in terms of the effectiveness in arresting bedwetting; the number of false alarms occurring; the life of the detector pad; the number of alarm breakdowns; the type of batteries, battery life, and the average cost of batteries per trial; and the effectiveness of the alarm in awakening the child in response to wetting episodes. The authors found that there were few differences between the various alarm systems with regards to the effectiveness in arresting bedwetting. However, most parents preferred the Eastleigh models and the Urilarm Deluxe models since these were found to result in fewer false alarms and fewer breakdowns, and the pads were more durable. While these observations are noteworthy, the authors conclude by commenting that their findings should not be taken to indicate a 'best buy' among the systems investigated because only a small number of children were allocated to each alarm group and other factors such as social conditions and the psychological state of the child were not controlled.

An American article by Mountjoy *et al.* (1984) sets out to address the topic of toilet training devices and the theoretical frameworks from which these have emerged. Of interest to the practitioner, the article includes a list of more than a dozen anti-enuretic devices commercially available in North America, together with details of manufacturers' addresses (and prices at the time). This list appears as Appendix 2 to the Mountjoy *et al.* article. Unfortunately, no attempt is made to evaluate these devices, some of which are for treating diurnal enuresis rather than bedwetting.

In Australia there are also several urine-alarm systems on the market. Five of these were evaluated in 1977 by *Choice*, a consumer protection magazine. The five brands were Drinite (Watson Victor Ltd, Australia), Eastleigh (United Kingdom), Instant Bell (Instant Bell Medical Equipment, Australia), Koowee (Sheereze, Australia), and Stop Wet (Practical Products, Australia). A striking finding of the *Choice* article was that none of the systems tested met the safety and operating requirements as set down the the British Ministry of Health's Performance Specifications for enuresis alarms. As a result, *Choice* felt unable to recommend any of the systems tested, although the Eastleigh apparatus came closest to the safety and operating requirements. The article concluded by urging the Standards Association of Australia to develop appropriate standards for the use of enuresis alarms.

The Eastleigh system
Of the bedwetting devices reviewed thus far, the Eastleigh system warrants special comment because it is easily the most commonly used apparatus. In their survey of 174 Health Authorities in the UK, the authors of the Oxford Regional Health report noted that 61% of all alarms in use carried the Eastleigh brand. Next most popular brands were the Wessex and Downs alarms which represented approximately 19% and 8% respectively of the alarms in use.

There are several Eastleigh systems in use but the one that features prominently in the recent literature is the Eastleigh MOH I, i.e. the transistorized version which conforms to the Ministry of Health specifications. This model consists of a robust alarm unit which is powered by a 6-volt battery and which emits a loud buzzing noise when triggered. There is a visual signal as well as an audio alarm. The alarm unit is connected to two mats made from specially woven anti-corrosive wire. The two mats are of different metallic composition and are bound at the edges with tape. Each mat is attached to the appropriate lead from the alarm unit by means of press studs.

Confidence in the reliability of equipment is a very important factor in retaining co-operation and enthusiasm for the conditioning treatment and the Eastleigh alarm has proven to be popular with therapists and parents of enuretic children because of its effectiveness in waking children following bed-wetting events, the infrequent incidence of false alarms and a low proportion of breakdowns. An additional advantage of the Eastleigh equipment is that is falls within a medium price bracket.

The most significant disadvantage of this model relates to the mats, which are inclined to curl up after a few weeks' usage, so that parents must straighten the meshes either by hand or by placing the mats under flat heavy objects. Furthermore, the effective lifespan of the mats is on average only about 3 months. While this is better than can be obtained with most other brands using the dual mat system, it is much shorter than the lifespan of the Coote pad described below. This problem is offset to some extent, however, by the relatively low cost in replacing the wire-meshed mats. Finally, it has been noted that, prior to becoming inoperable, the mats can lose sensitivity due to a deposit on the metallic gauze.

The Ramsey–Coote system

The major supplier of enuresis equipment in Australia over many years has been Ramsey–Coote Instruments. This system is a product of considerable research and development, including the treatment of thousands of bedwetters since 1954, and it is described in an article by Coote (1965). The system has been refined and modified over the years with advances in technology. The most unique feature remains the recessed-electrode bed-mat. This is a single rubber pad with moulded grooves into which are woven corrosion-resistant alloy braids. Unlike most models utilizing two mats, which are designed to serve the needs of a single case, and which consequently deteriorate fairly rapidly with constant use, the Ramsey–Coote mat is designed for multiple application. The accompanying alarm is also a very robust unit which triggers a loud bell and small fluorescent lamp in response to a bedwetting episode. The unit is driven by a permanently installed nickel cadmium battery and a small charger is supplied. There are outlet sockets for the optional accessories, i.e. the remote buzzer and the 'silent wakener', which is an almost noiseless, low frequency vibrator placed under the child's pillow. The silent wakener is useful for children who are difficult to arouse with conventional auditory signals, for cases with hearing impairments, for group situations (like dormitories, institutions, hospital wards and households where the enuretic child must share a bedroom with siblings), and for privacy of use in the case of mature-age bedwetters.

The major advantages of the Coote equipment are its reliability and durability. In busy enuresis clinics, where these devices are in use continuously, the pads have been known to have an effective lifespan of up to ten years, which is a much longer period than any of its competitors can claim. Also there are distinct advantages in single detector pads over the dual pad design. In general terms the Coote pad is easier to set up in the child's bed, moves around less and is more comfortable to sleep on.

The major disadvantage of the Coote equipment is its relatively high initial cost. The 1987 price in Australian currency for the complete unit (excluding accessories) was A$754.00, (A$517.00 for the alarm unit and A$237.00 for the pad alone). Clearly, for the clinician this initial outlay has to be weighed up against the potential demand on the equipment, its lifespan and the importance of reliability. More information about the Coote equipment can be obtained from Ramsey–Coote Instruments, 49 Ardoyne Street, Black Rock, Victoria 3193, Australia. There are plans to manufacture the Coote equipment under licence in the USA in the near future, and ultimately in Europe as well.

Another device currently available in Australia is manufactured by Cherub Industries, which is located at 41 David Terrace, Morphett Vale, South Australia, 5162. This consists of the alarm unit only which is designed to connect with the Coote pad. Features of the alarm include very high safety standards, a complex warbling signal when the alarm is triggered and rechargable batteries. The approximate cost of the Cherub alarm in 1988 is A$165.00.

We have used either the complete Ramsey–Coote or a combination of the Cherub alarm with the Coote pad in almost all of our clinical work which now totals approximately 2000 treatments. In general terms these systems have been highly effective. We are of the opinion that, in spite of its initial cost, there are definite advantages in the Coote pad because of its durability, efficiency and safety features. Furthermore, it is desirable to have more than one type of alarm signal for the large-scale treatment of bedwetting because some signals (e.g. a bell rather than a buzzer) are more effective in rousing some children than others.

2
Management

2.1 Initial investigations

MEDICAL

As already discussed when outlining the physiology of micturition in the previous chapter, it is actually quite rare for enuresis to be caused by organic disease. None the less, it is essential that before proceeding with treatment, every child identified as requiring treatment for nocturnal enuresis must first be examined by a medical practitioner, in order to determine whether or not there is any underlying organic disorder that could be the cause of the problem.

Initial medical investigation should include a detailed history, a measure of blood pressure, and the child's rate of growth for both height and weight, as this would be a marker for renal failure. Microscopic analysis of urine is essential and regarded as mandatory by most clinics with which we have been in contact. Additional radiologic and/or urologic investigations generally would not be required unless a physical abnormality was apparent from the initial checks, or the child failed to respond to treatment. If required, the first of these would most likely be an ultrasound examination of the renal tract. This is a non-invasive, safe method of obtaining a visual image of the organs involved in the urological system. Sometimes a special X-ray examination called an intravenous pyelogram (IVP) would be given. In this procedure a dye which acts as a contrast in the X-ray picture is injected into a vein and excreted by the kidneys. Thus, an outline of the collecting system of the kidneys, ureters and bladder is obtained.

The two other main investigations employed, especially to

determine whether or not the child has a neuropathic bladder, are a cystogram and a cystometrogram. In the former procedure, a dye is injected into the bladder and the bladder is then X-rayed as it empties. A normal bladder has smooth interior walls but a neuropathic bladder may have exaggerated folds and, sometimes, little pouches in it. A neuropathic bladder usually is larger than normal and the child is unable to empty it completely. Thus, the cystogram shows the amount of residual urine remaining in the bladder after voiding.

A cystometrogram measures bladder pressure. In this procedure, fluid is added to the bladder which is connected to a pressure meter. This method therefore effectively measures functional bladder capacity, i.e. the pressure of urine within the bladder that is required to trigger the chain of reflexes that culminate in voiding. Other accounts of the initial medical workup can be found in McKendry and Stewart (1974) and Jureidini (1982).

PSYCHOLOGICAL

Where the outcome of the medical investigation fails to establish a physical cause for enuresis and is therefore consistent with the bedwetting being functional in nature, it is necessary to conduct a psychological assessment before embarking on treatment. This usually would be done by a psychologist, using a structured interview involving the child, together with at least one parent.

Areas of interest include the child's history and pattern of bedwetting. Consistent with our position, expressed in section 1.1, about a possible association in some cases between emotional upset and bedwetting, we believe that it is important to determine whether the child is a primary or a secondary enuretic child and, in the case of the latter, to explore whether the onset of the enuresis appears to be associated with any personal, social or environmental circumstances which might have resulted in stress. It is also important to determine whether there is any pattern to the bedwetting (for example, whether the child wets only during the school week and not on weekends); and what is the overall frequency of bedwetting. The presence of other problems with continence, such as extensive urgency and/or frequency of micturition, or diurnal enuresis and encopresis, will help to determine what adjuvant therapies might be required. Any family history of enuresis, including any patterns of bedwetting among siblings and associated with either parent during their childhoods, should be explored. It has been noted already that there is a high incidence of childhood enuresis among parents, siblings and other near relatives of bedwetters and we have found that the identification of such a family history is frequently reassuring to the parents and enuretic child. This is because the history provides them with an explanation for the problem, which helps to dispel preconceived ideas about the problem being more sinister that it is in reality. At the same time the therapist must be careful to prevent the parents from developing any sense of guilt about responsibility for the problem. The parents' past attempts to curb the child's problem should also be discussed since such information can help the therapist to gain insight into the perceptions that the parents currently have about the nature and aetiology of enuresis. Clearly, where these are found to be inappropriate, then steps must be taken to redress this. We would note here that, occasionally, cases are encountered where the parents have already attempted treatment involving a bed-pad and alarm system, without success. Invariably, we have found it to be the case in such instances that either supervision in the use of this equipment has been lacking or inadequate, or that the equipment has been inferior. Thus, care is required when informing the child and the parents in this regard and in encouraging them to accept that, with adequate supervision and equipment, there are grounds for optimism about the outcome of treatment. In other words, what has been done in the past will influence the psychological preparation and supervision given by the therapist during treatment.

Although we would again emphasize, as already discussed in Chapter 1, that in most instances bedwetting is not caused by emotional disturbance, it is nevertheless the case that it can be accompanied by emotional and behavioural symptoms, which sometimes appear to be linked to specific educational or environmental circumstances. It is important, therefore, to assess the child's socio-emotional adjustment. Of particular interest are the child's school performance, peer group relationships and relationships with other family members. Specific fears that may be related functionally to bedwetting, such as fear of the dark or some toilet phobia, should also be identified. Most importantly, the child's own reaction to the enuresis, and the impact of this reaction on self-esteem and confidence and motivation to become dry, should be explored. If any of the above problems are uncovered, then they may need therapeutic intervention, in addition to the direct treatment of the bedwetting symptoms.

Accommodation arrangements should be reviewed. The location of the child's bedroom in relation to the toilet and the parents' bedroom, night-time lifting arrangements, the presence of siblings in the bedroom, and the general impact of the therapy programme on other members of the household, all need to be considered. These aspects of management are dealt with in more detail in section 2.3.

2.2 Psychological preparation for treatment

There are several reasons for emphasizing the importance of an adequate psychological preparation for both the enuretic child and the parents before treatment begins. In virtually every case, the parents and child will have already developed a set of preconceived notions about the nature and aetiology of enuresis as well as its treatment, and very often these beliefs are without foundation. It is most important, therefore, that an explanation for the nature of enuresis and a rationale for its treatment should dispel any misunderstandings that might be held about the problem. Secondly, as with any form of therapy the patient–therapist relationship is important, even though the therapeutic medium may be the application of specific stimulus conditions. At the very least, close contact between the therapist and the family helps to ensure adherence to the rules of the treatment programme, but regular contact is also valuable in maintaining the child's and parents' morale, while at the same time demonstrating a genuine interest in the child's welfare. Thirdly, the child's attitudes may need to be modified in order to obtain compliance with treatment. For example, the child may have fears and anxieties associated with what he or she believes is to follow and these need to be allayed before proceeding with treatment. Fourthly, there is now abundant evidence that bedwetting treatment that is not regularly supervised is much less effective than treatment involving a close degree of contact between the therapist and the family. Close supervision enables the therapist to detect equipment malfunction and errors of procedure more quickly, there is a greater opportunity for providing encouragement, and it has been found to reduce the rate of premature drop-out from treatment.

As a starting point to an interview with the family, we have found that it is worthwhile emphasizing the prevalence of enuresis in childhood. For adults and older children this can be achieved by providing average descriptive statistical information about incidence, like the 10–15% of five-year-olds and the 5% of ten-year-olds who wet the bed regularly. For younger children it is often beneficial to relate prevalence to the number of other bedwetters likely to be in their school on the basis of incidence. Thus, for children aged five to seven years (Junior Primary grades), it can confidently be said that there is likely to be at least one other bedwetter in the child's class. In an average primary school there may be altogether 20 or so children who wet the bed. Sometimes the enuretic child will know of other children who have a similar problem, and drawing attention to this can make it easier for the child to accept the problem. In cases where the child expresses doubts about the existence of other bedwetters, it can be pointed out that this may appear to be the case because it is the sort of problem that people often prefer not to disclose. Most children are quick to understand this point, since, almost always, they will have been very secretive about their own bedwetting.

The child and parents are typically reassured that, in the vast majority of cases, bedwetting does not reflect a sinister physical or emotional problem. (By this stage presumably the medical check will have been completed and the possibility of underlying organic pathology dismissed. Similarly, the therapist will have already had the opportunity of assessing the significance of any emotional factors and, indeed, whether these are primary or secondary to the problem.) Furthermore, the child can be strongly reassured that the treatment is painless and harmless and, provided that he/she co-operates, that the prospect of a cure is very high.

Next, an explanation of the problem should be made. We favour an explanation based on the notion that the bed-wetting results from a failure to learn to perceive the signals from a filling bladder during sleep and to respond appropriately, by contracting the bladder sphincter and/or by awakening to go to the toilet. An explanation to parents should be tailored to fit the parents' level of comprehension and, in most instances, a separate, less sophisticated explanation will be required for the child. As a general guide, we have found the following explanation, made with the aid of a simplified diagram of the bladder, to be useful for most children and their parents.

When we go to sleep our bladders continue to collect urine from our kidneys. This is quite normal. As the volume of urine increases, it puts pressure on the inside of our bladder, which then sends a message up to our brain. In order to avoid wetting the bed, our brain responds by telling the muscle at the opening of the bladder to tighten up. This is all automatic; it happens in our sleep without us being aware of it. None the less, as the bladder continues filling up, the muscle gets progressively tighter and usually we can hold on until the morning before having to go to the toilet. If the pressure inside our bladder becomes too great during the night, then the messages from the bladder to the brain tell us to wake up and to go to the toilet.

In the case of children who wet the bed, they have simply not learned this automatic bladder control. In other words, they go off to sleep and their bladders collect urine in the normal way, but they do not respond to the messages telling them to tighten the muscle at the bladder outlet, or to wake up. Consequently, when the pressure of urine reaches a certain point, the outlet to the bladder relaxes, resulting in a wet bed. The reasons for the child failing to learn the habit of keeping control over the bladder outlet vary and are still not fully understood. It is possible, for example, that the messages are not strong enough or that the child sleeps too deeply to perceive them.

In any event, to overcome bedwetting the object is to teach the child the habit of tightening the bladder outlet as required during sleep. This is done with the aid of the bed-pad and alarm device, which is an arrangement whereby a loud alarm is triggered as soon as the child wets. The sudden noise causes the child to close the bladder outlet tightly, and to relax the muscles which would otherwise squeeze the urine out of the bladder.

After the bedwetting accidents have been followed by the loud noise enough times, the child learns to tighten the bladder outlet before it begins to open. This stops the child from wetting and thereby avoids the noise. Eventually the child develops normal bladder control during sleep, without the aid of the bed-pad and alarm.

2.3 Practical treatment procedures

The following section is intended as a general model for the treatment procedure based on use of a bed-pad and alarm system. Of course, the procedure will need to be modified, to some extent at least, depending on specific situational factors, the familiarity of the parents and the child with the treatment programme, the design of the equipment, and so on. In almost all cases the treatment procedure can be demonstrated and followed up effectively from the therapist's office although, as will be seen from a case study to be described in section 3.4, there may be occasions when a visit to the family home is beneficial.

ESTABLISHMENT OF BASELINE

For at least two weeks prior to beginning treatment, the number of all bedwetting incidents and the nights during which they occur should be recorded carefully by a parent, in order to establish a baseline frequency of bedwetting, against which the effectiveness of subsequent treatment can be evaluated. This recording would usually be done between the initial assessment interview and the meeting which follows between the therapist and the child, together with at least one parent. The main object of this second meeting is to permit the therapist to demonstrate the treatment procedures and to instruct the child and parent in how to use the equipment, and more will be said about this below. It is advantageous to provide parents with a simple calendar or chart, appropriately set out so that recording is straightforward. It is emphasized to the parents that during this baseline period they must cease all pre-existing management procedures, such as waking or lifting during the night for toileting, imposing any fluid restrictions before bedtime, giving rewards for dry nights, or any form of punishment for wet nights.

DEMONSTRATION OF THE EQUIPMENT

There are now many different manufacturers of enuresis alarms, as already described in section 1.3 (p. 41). The equipment with which we are most familiar is that manufactured by Ramsey–Coote Instruments (Australia). However, while other brand names may vary from the Ramsey–Coote equipment in terms of the size and appearance of the instrument, the type of signal emitted and the electronic circuitry, the vast majority will consist of an alarm, together with a single urine-detector pad or a pair of mats. The detection device is placed in the child's bed and connected to the alarm which is operated by drycell batteries. These alternative arrangements are shown in Figure 2.1.

The urine-alarm equipment is demonstrated to the parents and child by pouring a small amount of sterile saline solution onto the detector pad, thereby triggering the alarm. The child is then encouraged to repeat this procedure, with one hand placed on the pad so as to reassure the child that there is no electric shock and nothing to fear from this equipment. Next, setting up the equipment is demonstrated, using a mock-up bed in the therapist's office. The bed is made up with a waterproof sheet to protect the mattress and, on top

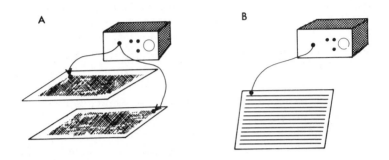

Figure 2.1 The bed-pad and alarm device; A illustrates the dual pad system; B illustrates the single pad system.

of the waterproofing, a normal linen sheet. Figure 2.2 illustrates this arrangement for both the single and double mat systems. The moisture-sensitive mat is positioned on top of the sheet so that it is underneath the child's buttocks when the child is lying normally. The mat is then covered by a cotton draw sheet, the edge of which should be tucked in firmly around the edge of the mattress. This reduces discomfort to the child and also helps to hold the pad in position throughout the night. Note that a nylon sheet is not suitable because this can encourage high perspiration. The child sleeps on top of the cotton draw sheet, covered by the normal bedding of top sheet, blankets, etc. The mat is connected to the alarm unit according to the instructions of the particular manufacturer. The alarm unit should be placed on a cupboard or side-table near the side of the bed but just beyond the child's reach, thereby requiring that the child get out of bed in order to turn off the alarm when it is triggered by a bedwetting event. At the same time, this arrangement ensures that the alarm is close enough to avoid loss of intensity in the signal. Equally, it is important to place the alarm on a hard surface, so that the signal will not be muffled when it sounds.

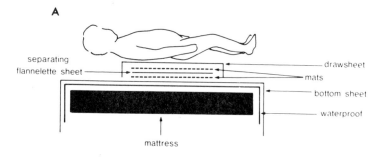

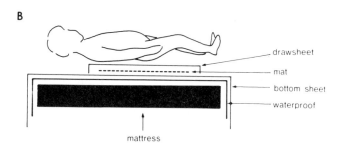

Figure 2.2 Method for laying out and assembling the bed-pad and
alarm device; A illustrates the dual pad arrangement;
B illustrates the single pad arrangement.

EXPLANATION OF THE STANDARD CONDITIONING METHOD

When the alarm is triggered in response to a bedwetting
episode, the child is required to do essentially three things.
The first is to get out of bed quickly and to turn off the
alarm. Secondly, the child is required to go to the toilet to
finish voiding, since, as treatment proceeds, the child will
retain more urine in the bladder (and pass less while in the
bed), and it is necessary to empty the bladder in order to
reduce the likelihood of subsequent accidents during the same

night. At least initially, it is advisable that a parent accompany the child to the toilet until this step has become established and the alarm should therefore be used to wake a parent, by integrating a separate alarm unit into the system and placing it in the parents' bedroom if that is necessary, or by arranging for a parent to sleep in the same room as the child for the first few nights. (The parent can also assist the child with the alarm resetting procedure if necessary.) The third step requires that the child should clean up the bed. He/she removes the wet draw sheet and wipes dry the rubber detector pad (or mats). Finally, a clean draw sheet is placed over the pad, the alarm is reset, and the child returns to sleep. It is advisable to have clean sheets in a convenient location on standby so that the child does not have to search for them in the middle of the night.

During training the child is required to role-play the three steps just described, using the demonstration bed, in order to ensure that the method for treatment has been understood. This whole routine is to be repeated every time that the child wets the bed and this requirement is emphasized with the child and with the parents. The child is encouraged to take full responsibility for the above steps, though parents will need to assist if the child is unable to manage alone. In cases where children need special motivation, as is sometimes the case with younger children, they can be encouraged to race their parents in reaching and turning off the alarm. Ordinarily, parental supervision will be required for the first few nights of training but this can be phased out quickly for most children over the age of about eight years of age, with the parents keeping only a cursory eye on things thereafter. The best attitude for parents to adopt is one of sympathetic help; that is, to give the impression that the bedwetting is a problem that both the parents and the child are going to work on together. However, we do encourage parents to maintain a discrete check on two aspects of the procedure that are absolutely essential to the successful progress of treatment. Firstly, a check must be made that the child has remembered to switch on the alarm at bedtime. Secondly, parents must check periodically that the batteries are 'alive' and adequate to sound the alarm whenever an accident occurs.

During treatment the child is encouraged to sleep without pyjama pants, in order to minimize the delay between voiding and triggering the alarm. However, if this is unacceptable to the child, it is usually possible to reach a compromise by having the child wear thin summer pyjamas. The child is encouraged to maintain a regular bedtime and, once a programme of treatment has begun, it is highly desirable to avoid any interruptions to the programme; for example, because of holidays or machine malfunction. It may be necessary to make special arrangements for the child to use night-lights to facilitate access to the toilet after a bedwetting incident. In addition, the proximity of the child's bedroom to the toilet is a consideration to be dealt with beforehand when discussing accommodation arrangements during treatment. Ideally, the child should be required to get out of bed and walk to the toilet, rather than finishing voiding in a pot placed in the bedroom. However, it is desirable to have easy access to the toilet. Similarly, it is advantageous for the parents to be in close proximity to the child's bedroom in order to supervise the procedure, especially in situations involving children who are young, or who do not wake readily to the alarm, and/or who are noncompliant.

During treatment it is rarely necessary to make special arrangements to separate the enuretic child from other children. However, if sleeping arrangements involve bunk beds, then the child being treated should be located in a lower bunk. Siblings sleeping in the same room may be disturbed during the first few nights but thereafter, in our experience, they seem relatively unaffected by the alarm. Indeed, we have successfully treated bedwetters in hospital wards, with only minimal disturbance to other patients. However, if siblings do complain about the noise in the normal domestic setting, then it is preferable to make special sleeping arrangements. Apart from any advantages to siblings, such arrangements will also tend to minimize social pressure on the enuretic child.

Written instructions for the treatment procedure and for

BEDWETTING ALARM – PROGRESS SHEET

NAME: Sophie

BASELINE: 14 Wet nights, 0 Dry

Date	Bedtime	Time awakened by alarm	Time of self awakening	Size of wet patch (large, medium, small)	Wet or Dry	Comments
START						
11.1.86	8-45	—	7-00 am	—	DRY	Great Start!
12.1.86	9-00	?	7-00 am	large (18")	WET	Turned off alarm and went back to sleep without going to toilet
13.1.86	9-00	2-00 am	7-15 am	v. small (3")	WET	
14.1.86	9-30	12-30 am	7-15 am.	medium (12")	WET	Had a late swim after dinner and seemed to be particularly tired.
15.1.86	9-00	10-00 pm	7-15am	medium (12")	WET	
16.1.86	9-00	12-45 am	7-15am	small (6")	WET	
17.1.86	10-30	7-45am	7-45am	medium (12")	WET	Slept in as it was week-end. Wet while waking up — Mother angry
19.1.86	10-30	—	8-00am	—	DRY	Hooray!!
19.1.86	8-30	10-30 pm 12-45 am	7-15 am	small (6") small (6")	WET	
20.1.86	9-00	—	6-00am	—	DRY	Hooray!! She woke early to make sure she was dry.
21.1.86	9-00	6-00am	6-00am	small (6")	WET	She wet again while waiting.
22.1.86	8-45	5-30 am.	7-30	v.small (3")	WET	Woke immediately in response to alarm
23.1.86	9-00	—	7-15	—	DRY	
24.1.86	10-30	12-30 pm	8-30	small (6")	WET	Disappointed — need reassurance.

Figure 2.3 The parents' record-keeping form

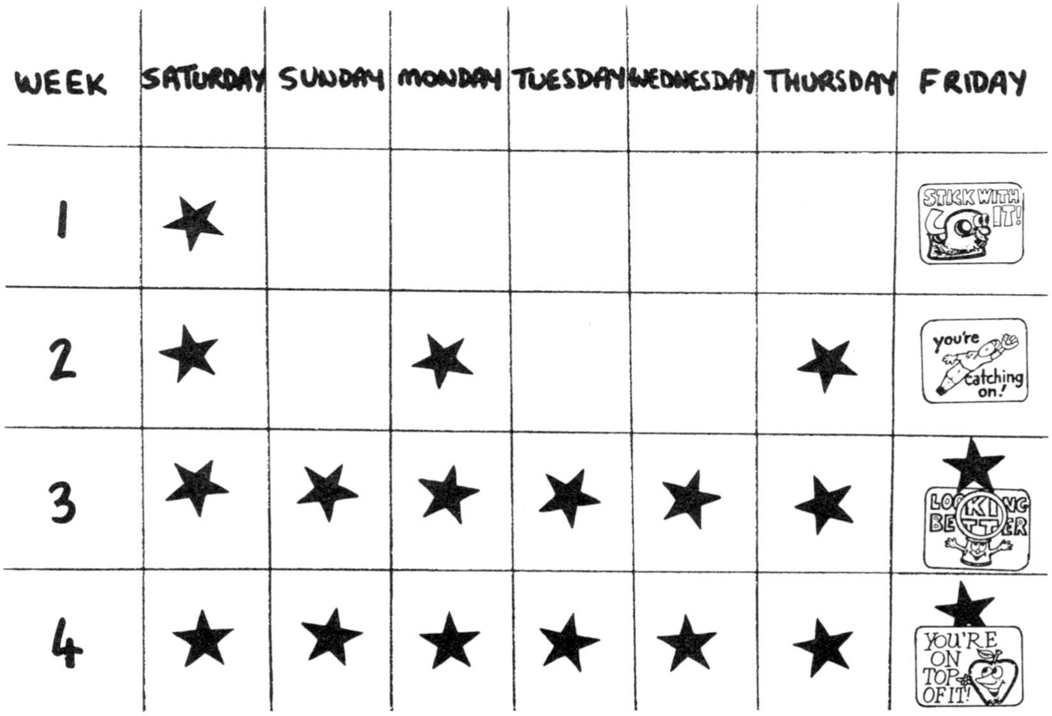

WEEK	SATURDAY	SUNDAY	MONDAY	TUESDAY	WEDNESDAY	THURSDAY	FRIDAY
1	★						STICK WITH IT!
2	★			★		★	you're catching on!
3	★	★	★	★	★	★	LOOKING BETTER
4	★	★	★	★	★	★	YOU'RE ON TOP OF IT!

Figure 2.4 The child's star chart record; a star indicates a dry night and blank cells signify a bedwetting event.

recording all bedwetting incidents are issued beforehand. The record form completed by the parents or older children provides more information than that used to establish baseline events. The example shown in Figure 2.3 was part of the record kept by the parents of Sophie, a nine-year-old girl whose treatment is described as the first case study in Chapter 3. The record shown here corresponds to the first four weeks of treatment summarized in Figure 3.1 (p. 87). As may be seen in Figure 2.3, the form requires that the parents collect daily information relating to the child's bedtime, the time at which the alarm is triggered, details of self-awakening for toileting, and an estimate of the size of the wet patch in the child's bed at the time when a bedwetting incident occurs. This last piece of information provides a rough index of the quantity of urine released. As will be discussed subsequently, the size of the patch can be used to monitor progress during treatment, even while the child is still continuing to wet the bed. Also, a column is provided on the form for any information regarding the programme that might be thought to be of interest to the therapist; (e.g. any incidents of machine malfunction, illness, interruptions to the programme due to holidays, instances of noncompliance, or failure to awaken in response to the alarm). Children under the age of about ten years can keep a separate record, in the form of a star chart, which can be drawn up with the therapist at the time of the instruction interview. Sophie's star chart for the first four weeks of treatment is included here as Figure 2.4.

Close supervision of the programme is essential since this supervision maintains progress, increasing the likelihood that the procedure is being followed correctly and providing support to both child and parents to persist with the programme. The importance of close supervision cannot be over-emphasized and, without it, a significant minority of parents may become disheartened and not persevere with the treatment procedures. Poor co-operation in this regard should not be regarded as reflecting parental indifference or unwillingness to help the child. The treatment programme can be disruptive to normal household routines and failures of equipment, which inevitably do occur sometimes, particularly because of loss of charge in the batteries, can be especially irritating. However, problems like the child not waking to the alarm initially, or of a false alarm because the mat was dried inadequately following an accident, or of an alarm failing to sound when an enuretic incident occurs because of a flat battery, can be anticipated on the basis of past experience and the parent and the child can therefore be alerted to these possibilities beforehand. Close supervision will certainly also help a family to cope with such problems.

The nature and frequency of the follow-up arrangements agreed upon will depend on a number of considerations, like the family's geographical location, the amount of time that the therapist can make available, and differences between families which emerge during interview in the need for support and guidance. However, as a general guideline that we believe has proven to be satisfactory in most cases, it is suggested that telephone contact once a week be maintained for progress reports, with a specific time for reporting being arranged with the parents or the child (if sufficiently mature) from the outset. In addition, if resources permit, it is desirable to schedule a personal visit by the child (together with a parent if necessary) to the therapist every four weeks or so. This arrangement is especially valuable for younger children who can present their star charts and, if reasonable progress has been made, be given a small reward. At the very least, on such occasions the parents and the child can be encouraged for their efforts. However, for some families living in remote areas, mail contact is probably the only practical means for staying in touch once the initial personal interview has taken place.

The detailed information recorded by the parents can be valuable for motivational reasons, as well as for guiding the therapist regarding any modifications of the programme that might be necessary. For example, with a child who wets the bed several times each night, it can be encouraging to begin with to observe that the size of the wet patch is diminishing over time, or that the accidents are occurring further into the night, even though a completely dry night has not yet been achieved. In addition, the parents and therapist may observe patterns in the child's wetting habits which may influence the precise form of therapeutic intervention developed – such as an association between bedtime and accidents, a failure to respond to the alarm, or proneness to accidents only on school days.

Parents are encouraged to contact the therapist immediately if any difficulties arise before the designated weekly contact time. It is essential, too, that any case who does not report at the designated time or who fails to attend a meeting, be contacted immediately by the therapist in order to update the child's progress. In the event of persistent failure to comply with contact requirements it may become necessary to discontinue treatment although, in our experience, such cases are rare.

We recommend that treatment should continue until the child has achieved at least 14 consecutive dry nights, completely free from any bedwetting episode but of course this criterion, although now commonly adopted, is an arbitrary one. There are no hard and fast rules about the termination of treatment and in much of our work we have actually preferred to use a criterion of 21 consecutive dry nights, and even 28 and more with some cases. As a rule of thumb, a longer criterion period does permit a greater confidence that a complete remission will be achieved. However, the target of 14 consecutive dry nights has become the conventional success criterion in many recent experimental studies with a urine-alarm system and, on balance, this appears to be satisfactory in most cases. The criterion applied will also be influenced by the availability of equipment and by the need to 'turn over' urine-alarms in clinics where there is a large demand for their use. At least for most cases, 14 consecutive dry nights will be achieved by between ten to twelve weeks of treatment and this will herald eventual permanent nocturnal continence for most children. In our experience, progress at about this rate does not unduly hold up the acquisition of a bed-pad and alarm for the next child on a clinic waiting list. However, in some instances alternative success criteria will need to be established. For example, a child who wets infrequently or sporadically may need to demonstrate a longer period of continence before treatment is terminated. Additionally, some children become dependent on the alarm, or at least come to see it as a form of security. In such cases it is advisable, together with appropriate reassurance, to remove the bed-pad and alarm from the child's bed after the child has achieved the dryness criterion but to keep the apparatus in the home until a further seven consecutive dry nights have been achieved.

If little progress has been made after about four months of treatment, then the child's treatment should be reviewed by the therapist. In such cases a break from therapy might be tried before resuming later, and a further medical review should also be considered.

In light of the high relapse rate following initial success with the standard conditioning procedure, it is advisable to meet in person with the child and parents at the completion of treatment, rather than have them simply return the equipment without meeting. This meeting provides an opportunity for warning the child and the parents that relapse is a fair possibility while, at the same time, reassuring them that subsequent treatment is readily available should this turn out to be necessary. However, a careful distinction should be drawn between isolated or very occasional wetting accidents, that may occur for some months after the achievement of a long initial period of dryness, and a genuine relapse where frequent bedwetting becomes re-established. It will generally be possible to link occasional accidents to instances of exhaustion, illness, or some important change in the child's routine. On the other hand, relapse is, by definition, a resumption of regular bedwetting – for example, wetting more than once a week throughout a period of several weeks. Similarly, treatment may sometimes be followed by sporadic lapses, but without any trend or consistent wetting pattern becoming established. In such cases, it is best initially to reassure the child if necessary but to otherwise ignore the problem. However, discussion with the parents should emphasize that, should it become clear that a true relapse has occurred, then they should contact the therapist without delay. In this event a second trial using the bed-pad and alarm will be necessary but, even so, the parents and child can be reassured that the second treatment is usually quicker to succeed than the first, and more durable. Only a small minority of children have multiple relapses – perhaps as few as 10% of all cases of relapse. None the less, the problem of relapse following conditioning treatment is significant and, because of this, there is merit in warning parents at the commencement of treatment of the possibility that the child may need two (or in very rare cases more) trials using the bed-pad and alarm apparatus before complete success is achieved.

2.4 Adjuvant therapies

It has been argued in earlier sections that, for the majority of enuretic children, bedwetting represents a learning or habit deficiency involving a failure to achieve control over the bladder sphincter during sleep. For these children the standard conditioning procedure involving the bed-pad and alarm is usually efficient and effective in clearing up the problem. However, in any large group of enuretic children, one finds considerable variability in terms of bedwetting frequency, ease of arousability from sleep, functional bladder capacity, the presence of day-time symptoms, motivation to become dry, and so on. Thus, depending on the child's particular needs, it is often beneficial to supplement the treatment procedure based on the bed-pad and alarm with other strategies that have been shown to help to reduce bedwetting in some cases. The most common of these are now described.

WAKING SCHEDULE

It is common practice among parents of bedwetters to awaken the child during the night for toileting and many parents report that this is effective in reducing bedwetting frequency somewhat, although the practice does not commonly lead to a wholly effective cure. Thus, if in such cases the practice of waking the child is discontinued, then it is very likely that a higher frequency of bedwetting will resume immediately.

Empirical evidence for the effectiveness of waking programmes as a therapeutic strategy is limited by the small
number of studies reported and, with one or two exceptions,
by the small number of subjects in each study. However, one
of the most detailed and systematic waking schedules is
employed in Dry-Bed Training (Azrin *et al.* 1974). According
to Azrin *et al.* (1974), this procedure helps to develop the
ease with which the enuretic child can be aroused from sleep,
by providing the child with regular practice at having to
rouse quickly during the night. The schedule also includes a
requirement that the parents progressively reduce the amount
of prompting necessary to rouse the child, thereby gradually
shaping self-initiated waking. It is also likely that the waking
schedule creates more opportunities for positive reinforcement by parents in the form of praise and other forms of
social reward, as a consequence of the child maintaining a
dry bed. Positive reinforcement is given at the time of each
scheduled awakening when the child is required to feel the
sheets and is praised for keeping them dry. In addition,
requiring the child to empty the bladder on each occasion
when he/she is awakened increases the probability that the
child will remain dry throughout the night and, for each such
occasion, will therefore result in further positive reinforcement on the following morning.

Because of its general utility, as already discussed when
describing Dry Bed Training in Chapter 1 (p. 34), the full
waking   schedule   taken   from   the   Dry-Bed   Training
programme is now described here in some detail. This
schedule is designed to provide training in three stages. The
first (Part 1) is the All-night training session, carried out for
the initial night only. Azrin *et al.* (1974) have recommended
that this session be supervised by a professional trainer who
spends the night at the enuretic child's home but, as
described   above,   we   have   established   that,   following
appropriate instruction, the child's parents can supervise this
training very effectively. Part 2 starts the following night and
describes how a parent should wake the child at various
times throughout the night, according to a special, variable
waking schedule, the changes in which reflect any progress as

the child begins to achieve dry nights. Part 3 then begins when the child has reached a criterion of seven consecutive dry nights.

Part 1: All-night training

STEP A: AT BEDTIME

1. The all-night trainer (either the therapist or a parent) sets up the bed-pad and alarm according to a detailed instruction sheet which outlines how to remake the child's bed with the pad in place, where the alarm should be located, and how the alarm is switched on and connected to the pad. A copy of these instructions is included in the Appendix.
2. The trainer explains what will be happening to the child; that is, that tonight he/she will be awakened every hour to practise going to the toilet and that if he/she wets, he/she will have to change the bedsheets and go to the toilet again.
3. The child then goes to sleep.

STEP B: HOURLY AWAKENINGS

1. Throughout the first night the child is awakened each hour by the trainer and is sent or is accompanied to the toilet. The child is awakened, using as little prompting as possible. Thus, if necessary on the first occasion, the child is helped to sit up in bed and gently shaken if not completely awake. On the next occasion the trainer might try just shaking the child gently on the shoulder, without actually helping him/her to sit up. The idea is to reduce on each occasion the things that the trainer needs to do in order to wake the child. In this way the child will gradually learn to get up without help. The bedroom light is not turned on unless this is really necessary. If the child does not go straight to the toilet on wakening, the trainer points towards the toilet and asks 'Where do you go when I wake you up?' If the child still does not walk towards the toilet, the trainer takes him/her quickly into the toilet saying, 'You have to *hurry* to the toilet if you don't want to wet your bed.'

2. After returning from the toilet the child gets back into bed.
3. At this time the trainer asks the child if the bedsheets are dry and encourages the child to feel the sheets and to tell the trainer that they are dry.
4. The trainer then praises child for having a dry bed and encourages him/her to keep it dry for the next hour.
5. Before returning to sleep the child is asked to repeat the training instructions which describe what he/she is to do for the next hourly toileting.
6. The child then returns to sleep.

STEP C: WHEN THE CHILD WETS THE BED
1. The trainer wakes the child and gives a brief, mild reprimand.
2. The trainer turns off the bedwetting alarm if the child has not already done so.
3. The trainer sends the child to the toilet to finish urinating.
4. The child is now given cleanliness training, requiring that he/she
   (a) changes into clean pyjamas;
   (b) removes the wet draw sheet from the bed, wipes the rubber pad dry and puts the wet draw sheet into the laundry;
   (c) remakes the bed (with parental assistance if necessary) by covering the rubber pad with a dry draw sheet.
5. The trainer switches the bedwetting alarm on again.
6. The child returns to sleep.

Part 2: For nights following the initial all-night training

STEP A: AT BEDTIME
1. The bedwetting alarm is set.
2. A parent reminds the child of the need to remain dry and tells him/her that if a wetting accident occurs then he/she will have to go through the cleanliness training routine (as set out for Step C, point 4, under the all-night training procedure above).
3. The parent asks the child to repeat all instructions so that

the parent can be sure that the child has understood and remembers them.

STEP B: THE WAKING SCHEDULE
1. A parent awakens the child about three hours after the child has gone to bed and sends him/her to the toilet.
2. After each dry night, the parent awakens the child 30 minutes earlier than on the previous night.
3. This waking procedure continues until the scheduled time for waking is within one hour from the child's bedtime. At this point, waking the child is discontinued.

STEP C: ACCIDENTS
If the child wets the bed, then the parent gives him/her the cleanliness training immediately. On the following night the waking schedule returns to the first step, where the child is awakened three hours after going to bed.

STEP D: AFTER A DRY NIGHT
1. The parents should praise the child for not wetting the bed.
2. The parents also encourage other relatives (where this is possible) to praise the child for not wetting.
3. Members of the family praise the child again, at least five times during the day, using every opportunity, like during meals, or just before bedtime, etc.

Part 3: Normal routine
This begins when the child has accomplished seven dry nights in a row.

1. The bed-pad is removed from the bed, together with the alarm. This can be done by the child, under parental supervision to guard against any damage to the equipment.
2. A parent inspects the child's bed each morning and records whether it is wet or dry and, if wet, the size of the patch. The child is encouraged to do this also.
3. If the child wets on two nights in the one week, then the parents goes back to Part 2 (i.e. the night after initial training) and maintains that regimen until the child has

again reached seven consecutive dry nights. When this is achieved training returns to Part 3 (i.e. the normal routine).
4. Treatment is regarded as completed when the child has achieved a further seven dry nights in a row – that is, 14 consecutive dry nights in all.

As described in Chapter 1, a study by Bollard and Nettelbeck (1981) showed that a combination of the waking schedule described above with the urine-alarm was virtually as effective in arresting bedwetting as the complete Dry-Bed Training programme. For practical purposes, this finding is of considerable advantage because of the demands of the full programme. The waking schedule itself presents additional demands to the standard conditioning method but these are not substantial other than during the initial night of training when the child is awakened hourly for toileting. Thus, it is recommended that, in the case of a child who is particularly difficult to rouse in response to the standard bed-pad and alarm procedure during the first few weeks of treatment, the waking schedule described above should be added to the alarm procedure. Indeed, since the waking schedule is not excessively demanding, and in many cases amounts to nothing more than what the parents have already been doing prior to the commencement of organized treatment, it could be recommended that the waking schedule be incorporated in the standard conditioning programme from the outset for virtually all enuretic children undergoing treatment.

RETENTION CONTROL TRAINING

There is evidence that, on average, the enuretic child does have a smaller functional bladder capacity than nonenuretic children of the same age. This has been determined by measuring the amount of urine passed at each voiding, and from the frequency of micturition measured over a fixed period of time. Generally, no difference is found between enuretic and nonenuretic children with respect to the total amount of urine passed, either during the day or night.

Furthermore, it has been found that the bladder volume of enuretic children under a general anaesthetic is comparable with that found among nonenuretic children under similar circumstances. However, among enuretic children the average number of voidings per 24 hours is significantly higher and the average volume of urine at each voiding is therefore significantly lower. Thus, while there is usually no intrinsic abnormality in the bladder of enuretic children which prevents the accommodation of normal quantities of urine, such children may tend to have smaller functional bladder capacity. It is worth noting, however, that this inference is made from comparisons between enuretic and nonenuretic groups. In so far as the treatment of individual cases is concerned, a decision about whether low functional bladder capacity is involved or not is difficult. This is because, to this time, there are no well-established age-related norms for functional bladder capacity. Moreover, the methods for measuring such capacity are far from precise and the procedures involving a general anaesthetic are obviously too invasive to be generally applied.

Increases in functional bladder capacity have been found to correlate positively with decreased bedwetting. Early attempts to treat enuresis by increasing functional bladder capacity frequently involved the use of a mechanical device to raise the neck of the bladder, thereby allowing more urine to be stored. However, these days most treatments aimed at increasing functional bladder capacity use increased fluid intake to achieve this end and this method has become known as **retention control training**.

Essentially, retention control training is a day-time procedure which involves, first, increasing the child's fluid intake and then, secondly, requiring that the child withholds voiding for as long as possible. The withholding time is gradually increased across each of several successive days and positive reinforcement is given for increased fluid intake and, again, immediately following each successful attempt at increasing the interval over which this fluid is retained. The effectiveness of retention control training by itself as a treatment for bedwetting is questionable since trials have met with mixed success, with earlier studies before about 1973 appearing to show more optimistic results than studies done since that time. None the less, it is our opinion that retention control training can be an effective supplement to the bed-pad and alarm procedure for enuretic children who display one or more of the following features:

1. Excessive frequency of voiding during the day or night.
2. Urgency of micturition; i.e. when the child apparently receives little warning of the need to void and often has to make a last minute dash to the toilet, only to have a wetting accident along the way.
3. The presence of diurnal enuresis, particularly when this involves frequent wetting episodes and often with only a small amount of urine being passed in the child's pants.
4. Difficulty in starting and/or stopping the urinary stream when voiding in the toilet. This may indicate, first, that only a low volume of fluid is being stored and there may therefore be only a low pressure of urine in the bladder; and, secondly, poor control of the abdominal and perineal muscles that are involved in starting and stopping the urinary stream at will.

The following steps are suggested as a model for retention control training, to be used as an adjunct to the bed-pad and alarm procedure.

1. Each day after the child has returned home from school, the child should be required to void in the toilet and then to have a large drink of anything palatable to the child and acceptable to the parent. The volume of fluid will vary, depending on the child's physical size and on individual differences in respect of the amount of fluid intake that can be tolerated. However, the following specifications provide a reasonable guideline. Children weighing less than 25 kilograms (kg) should drink 30 millilitres (ml) of fluid per kilogram of body weight, to a maximum of 500 ml. Those children weighing more than 25 kg should receive 20 ml of fluid per kilogram of body weight, to a maximum of one litre.
2. After drinking, the child is urged to refrain from voiding

for as long as possible. The child can engage in any activity during this period of 'holding on'. When the child insists that it is not possible to hold on any longer, he/she is required to void in the toilet and the period for which fluid was retained – i.e. the time between the initial fluid intake and subsequent voiding – is recorded on a chart.

3. This procedure of 'holding on' is repeated once only each day. On weekends and holidays a time for the retention control training is chosen that will be convenient for the child and for the family as a whole. Each day the child is encouraged to hold on longer than was accomplished on the previous day, by about an additional two minutes.

4. Positive reinforcement in the form of praise or some other reward is given when the child succeeds in increasing fluid intake and immediately following each successful attempt at lengthening the retention interval. Eventually the child will reach a maximum retention interval – recognizable because performance will become relatively stable from day to day – and at this point the child is reinforced for maintaining the same interval.

5. In addition to the retention training, the child is encouraged to practise starting and stopping the urinary stream when voiding. This can be done at any time that the child uses the toilet. Practice in stopping the urinary stream is useful in strengthening the perineal muscles in the crutch, which raises the bladder neck and tighten the internal sphincter. Starting the stream helps to develop the ability to push down the thoracic wall and to tighten the abdominal muscles.

6. This overall procedure is continued until the child reaches the dryness criterion, which commonly is 14 consecutive dry nights. Retention control training is not a particularly demanding adjunct to the bed-pan and alarm procedure but, nevertheless, it will require support and encouragement from both the parents and the therapist.

POSITIVE PRACTICE AND SOCIAL MOTIVATION

It is not uncommon when following the standard bed-pad

and alarm procedure for the enuretic child to lose the motivation to persist with the programme, particularly if the training turns out to extend over a long period of time. The average duration of treatment to secure continence by this method is about 10–12 weeks, a period of time involving a demanding schedule and certainly sufficiently long to test the motivation of many children and their families. Furthermore, in some cases, the child may actually be actively noncompliant from the outset of treatment, which most typically has been sought by the parents on the child's behalf. In most cases, such problems can be overcome by placing a greater emphasis on the system of rewards and punishment, on social motivation factors, and by the therapist maintaining close contact and supervision of the treatment programme, as already discussed above when describing the standard bed-pad and alarm procedure. However, on occasions when non-compliance or poor motivation persists, a supplementary procedure called **positive practice** (taken from the Dry-Bed Training programme) may be worthwhile.

Positive practice is derived from a technique called **over-correction** which is intended to decrease the incidence of undesirable behaviour, while simultaneously providing instruction to assist in the learning of a more adaptive form of response. Thus, the rationale is to educate the child by way of procedures which require that he/she replaces the unacceptable behaviour with behaviour for which approval can be shown. Once behaviour has improved, then 'massed practice' of appropriate behaviour is organized in the situation in which the undesirable behaviour previously occurred.

Over the past decade, numerous studies employing over-correction have appeared in the literature and, in most of the published reports, this approach has been found to be highly effective in modifying behaviour. The types of undesirable target behaviour studied have included aggression on the part of the child, self-stimulation, self-injury, vomiting, public disrobing, stealing, nervous habits and tics, and encopresis. Over-correction has also been used successfully as part of day-time toilet-training programmes for profoundly retarded adults and nonretarded young children. Over-correction is already a component in the standard bed-pad and alarm procedure, in so far as the child is normally required to change the wet sheets and to deposit them in the laundry, and then to re-make the bed in response to wetting episodes. Positive practice involves the additional requirement that the child practices going to the toilet several times following each bedwetting episode.

The specific steps of positive practice are that, after the child has completed the procedures of toileting and re-making the bed in response to a wetting episode, he/she should;

1. lie in bed with the light off; count up to 50, slowly and silently.
2. The child then gets up and goes to the toilet and tries to urinate.
3. The child returns to bed.
4. The child repeats steps (1) to (3) until this has been done a specified number of times.

This procedure is repeated every time a bedwetting episode is detected. During positive practice, the parents should stay out of the room but try to keep a check on the number of trips that the child makes to the toilet. The requirement that the child should count to 50 and repeat visits to the toilet 20 times has generally been followed for children over the age of eight years. For younger children the requirement has generally been to count to 20 and repeat the visit to the toilet eight times.

It has been our experience that parents and children find positive practice to be the most tedious and demanding component of bedwetting treatment. It is very time-consuming, and enforcement of the procedure sometimes invokes hostility on the part of the child and increases family tension, so that negative reactions from both parents and child to this requirement are not uncommon. The child sometimes manifests his/her anger by refusing to do the full complement of positive practice trials and, in addition, many parents express concern about having to administer such aversive procedures with their children. When these reactions occur it would seem sensible to drop the positive practice requirement from the treatment programme, since we have found gains associated with the procedure appear to be relatively modest.

However, notwithstanding the above observations, positive practice can be a worthwhile adjunct to the bed-pad and alarm procedure if children are poorly motivated and/or noncompliant. Thus, positive practice can usefully be employed at the beginning of treatment if the child is not highly motivated, to help to establish the required toileting regimen. We have also found positive practice to be useful following periods where the child's compliance with the treatment procedure wavers.

2.5 Management of relapse

While the effectiveness of treatment procedures for bed-wetting based on the bed-pad and alarm equipment is well established, a high probability of subsequent relapse remains a disappointing shortcoming of these procedures. A very wide range of relapse rates have been reported in the literature on this topic (Doleys, 1977), principally because, as with the estimation of the prevalence of bedwetting, there is no general consensus regarding what constitutes a relapse. Some researchers have regarded any renewed wetting as sufficient evidence that relapse has occurred, whereas other definitions have ranged as high as three wet nights within a week, or have been based on additional considerations, like a return to a level of bedwetting sufficient to cause parents to seek retreatment. Other difficulties in defining relapse are related to the duration of the follow-up period applied, with longer follow-up periods tending to be associated with higher rates of relapse; yet another problem arises from variation among studies in the percentage of cases treated who are subsequently followed up. However, despite such difficulties, as a general working rule it can be expected that, following an initial successful treatment, somewhere between about 30–40% of children will recommence wetting the bed sufficiently frequently to require follow-up treatment. If a child remains dry for six months following treatment, then the probability of a relapse is greatly reduced. None the less, some relapses do occur as long as two years after treatment and, furthermore, a small number of cases may require multiple treatment trials before a cure is achieved. One such case has been described in some detail in section 3.6.

Various attempts have been made to develop predictors or response to conditioning therapy, including subsequent relapse, but no particular clinical or treatment variable has yet been found to be definitely associated with the probability of relapse, although there is some evidence that where the period of treatment before achieving dryness is relatively short, then the likelihood of relapse is increased. This finding may be of particular significance for those situations where central nervous system stimulants like Methedrine and Dexedrine have been prescribed as an adjunct to conditioning treatment involving a bed-pad and alarm, since results from studies of this kind have generally found that the initial arrest of bedwetting has occurred significantly earlier with cases where drugs have been used in conjunction with an alarm method, that where an alarm procedure alone has been followed. Consistent with this suggestion, such studies have also generally found that the frequency of relapses was significantly higher among subjects to whom Dexedrine had been administered, compared with children treated by the alarm procedure but without drugs being included as part of the treatment.

It has also been found that if a child wets the bed frequently, and particularly if he/she also suffers from diurnal urgency and/or from frequency of micturition, then a relapse of bedwetting following treatment is more likely. More generally, there has also been some indication that children with diurnal symptoms are likely to relapse earlier than children with no day-time problems.

COUNTERMEASURES TO RELAPSE

Countermeasures to relapse following treatment by a bed-pad

and alarm procedure have generally followed one or both of two strategies; first, using the alarm in an **intermittent schedule** of presentation so that the alarm is activated in accordance with a predetermined percentage of wetting incidents (for example, the alarm rings following 50% of bedwets, according to a fixed ratio schedule); and, secondly, **overlearning**, whereby the child's fluid intake before bedtime is increased, particularly towards the end of treatment.

Intermittent reinforcement
An intermittent reinforcement schedule is one where the alarm is set to ring following a fixed percentage (e.g. 50%) of bedwetting incidents. Some researchers have designed special alarm equipment that automatically provides the schedule decided upon. However, an easy, practical means of achieving an intermittent schedule when using a standard alarm is simply to randomly select beforehand those nights when the alarm is not set to sound and then to instruct the child and parents accordingly. Obviously, written directions are desirable in such cases.

In accordance with his theoretical formulation of the standard bed-pad and alarm treatment as an avoidance learning paradigm, as opposed to classical conditioning, Lovibond (1964) proposed that an intermittent reinforcement procedure could be employed to reduce relapse by, in effect, reducing the likelihood that appropriate avoidance responding would become extinguished once the child had reached the dryness criterion and had therefore been taken off the alarm. Some studies following this suggestion have found that intermittent procedures produce significantly fewer relapses, while at the same time being as effective in arresting bedwetting as continuous reinforcement (i.e. the standard procedure where the alarm follows every bedwetting incident). It is by no means the case, however, that the intermittent reinforcement technique always successfully overcomes the problem of relapse and, at this time, no explanation can be given as to why this is so. Virtually nothing is known about the relative effectiveness of different kinds of fixed ratio schedules, although there are suggestions in the literature that a higher schedule of alarm usage (e.g. 70 per cent) may be more effective than, say, 50 per cent. Nor is it the case that marker characteristics can be used to identify those cases where an intermittent alarm schedule is likely to prove useful in combating relapse. Essentially, the therapist is in the position of waiting to see if relapse occurs and, if so, experimenting with intermittent schedules (or other procedures, to be discussed below) as a means of addressing this problem.

Overlearning

Overlearning training involves increased fluid intake and therefore bears similarities to the retention control procedure described earlier in this chapter. The overlearning procedure was first adopted by Young and Morgan (1972) and, essentially, it requires that the child first achieves the initial success criterion of, for example, 14 consecutive dry nights. From that point on, each night the child must drink a large volume of extra fluid – up to the maxima recommended under the retention control procedure already described above – preferably during the last hour before going to bed for the night. It is this increase in fluid, and the circumstances which accompany it, that is held to be responsible for the overlearning.

According to Morgan (1978) there are probably several principles involved. Firstly, the increase in fluid intake places increased demands on newly acquired responses assumed to underlie the reduction in the incidence of bedwetting. Thus, these demands either demonstrate a 'margin of error' in the learning already acquired (if it is the case that no further wetting episodes occur) or, where wetting is renewed, they afford further learning trials. Secondly, overlearning may increase the child's confidence to control the bladder at night through successively testing out this ability, although there must be some doubt about this as an explanation. Thus, simply extending the length of the success criterion, without increasing fluids, might also be seen as a means of increasing confidence, but this kind of extension to the success criterion does not seem particularly effective on its own in reducing the likelihood of relapse. The more effective control that accompanies overlearning may therefore be more a function of increased functional bladder capacity which, as we have already pointed out, some authors have suggested is a central factor in the successful treatment of bedwetting.

Research has suggested that both an intermittent alarm procedure and overlearning accompanied by the bed-pad and alarm are superior to the unaccompanied standard conditioning treatment of bedwetting, with respect to reducing subsequent relapse; and that a composite procedure of overlearning with bed-pad and alarm is superior to intermittent reinforcement. However, both intermittent reinforcement and overlearning procedures are known to increase the time required to attain the dryness criterion. The only study to compare the standard bed-pan and alarm procedure with intermittent reinforcement and overlearning method directly (Taylor and Turner, 1975) showed a clear difference in acquisition time, the durations of treatment before continence was achieved being 68, 113 and 86 days respectively for each of these procedures. Thus, intermittent reinforcement and overlearning may decrease relapse but at the cost of extending initial treatment considerably. These procedures may therefore introduce new problems within large enuresis clinics, where staff resources are usually not sufficient to meet the heavy extent of contact that becomes necessary to maintain a treatment programme in which noncompliance problems have accompanied extended treatment; or where the average time spent in treatment is the critical factor in determining the future availability of equipment for children already on a waiting list.

LONG-TERM EFFECTS OF DRY-BED TRAINING

Research has demonstrated that, on average, the Dry-Bed Training procedure can achieve an initial arrest of bedwetting more quickly than the standard bed-pad and alarm method, which is not accompanied by the various adjunctive procedures. However, as already discussed in preceding sections, the gains are not necessarily as marked as earlier research suggested they might be. Similarly, most recent research suggests that Dry-Bed Training does not result in a lower rate of subsequent relapse than the standard procedure, although it had been expected that the various training features of Dry-Bed Training in addition to the urine-alarm could operate in combination with one another to facilitate permanent nocturnal bladder control.

3
Case studies

We have selected the following cases of nocturnal enuresis to represent the wide spectrum of differences between individual children that a clinician might expect to encounter in the course of normal practice. Most of these cases have been drawn from among children treated recently in an enuresis clinic at a large metropolitan children's hospital, with the rest being from among children treated by the first author on a private basis. In all cases, the therapist referred to is one or other of us, but for those cases drawn from the enuresis clinic, treatment has involved substantial support from technical and ancillary staff connected with the clinic. We would emphasize that, while the range of problems here represents a broad sample of the enuretic population, the problems described do not occur with equal frequency. In fact, by far most of the cases treated within such a setting will involve either primary enuresis, a problem with waking readily to the alarm, or noncompliance with treatment procedures by either the child or parents and other members of the family.

3.1 Treating a primary enuretic child

This case is presented first because the girl involved represents a typical example of primary nocturnal enuresis in terms of her history, the presentation of the problem and the girl's response to treatment. The patient was nine years old. We will call her Sophie, although, of course, that is not her real name. She had two older siblings, her father was a self-employed accountant and her mother was engaged in home duties, supplemented by casual office work to assist the father in his business. The family enjoyed a comfortable middle-class lifestyle. As is often the case, bedwetting was not the principal reason for which Sophie had been referred to a psychologist. She had actually been referred because of concern on the part of her parents about her school progress and it was only during the course of an investigation into the nature of her learning difficulties that her bedwetting was uncovered.

The developmental history in this case revealed that Sophie had achieved all milestones at age-appropriate stages, with the exception of nocturnal bladder control. Toilet training for diurnal bladder and bowel control had been achieved without fuss by the time she was about two years of age. However, she had never mastered nocturnal bladder control and had wet the bed almost every night of her life. As a pre-schooler Sophie had exhibited urinary frequency and urgency during the day and she had had the occasional wetting accident, although these symptoms had not created a significant management problem and they did not continue after she had started at school. Earlier comprehensive medical examinations had failed to detect evidence of any underlying organic disease.

The parents had attempted a variety of strategies in the past to arrest Sophie's bedwetting. These had included fluid restriction following the evening meal, waking and lifting during the night for toileting, reward systems for dry nights and a trial on medication (imipramine). Furthermore, Sophie had had a previous trial on a bed-alarm device, which her parents had hired from a local pharmacy. However, this device had proved to be unreliable and had not been effective in waking Sophie at the time of bedwetting events. Moreover, no supervision of this treatment programme had been provided; the parents had simply been issued with the alarm, together with a set of very basic instructions, and left to their own resources. They had been charged a weekly rental fee for the equipment and instructed to return the alarm when the child stopped wetting the bed.

All of the above strategies for treatment had been unsuccessful. The parents had never punished Sophie for wetting the bed and in general they had not over-reacted to the problem. However, now that Sophie was nine years of age, both she and her parents were becoming anxious to arrest the problem.

During the course of the initial assessment interview, Sophie impressed as being an outgoing, socially well-adjusted child. She admitted to being bothered by her bedwetting, particularly since it prevented her from sleeping overnight at friends' houses. Similarly, she was somewhat bothered by her learning difficulties but otherwise she enjoyed school and had many friends. Her parents were caring and supportive and relationships within the family appeared to be healthy. It was noteworthy that the parents regarded Sophie as being an exceptionally deep sleeper. In addition, there was a significant family history of enuresis, in that the mother had been a bedwetter herself until the age of 14 years, when all bedwetting had ceased spontaneously.

In Sophie's case, initial management involved a psychometric assessment of here educational problems. Results of the Wechsler Intelligence Scale for Children (WISC-R) showed her level of general intelligence to fall within normal limits and there were no specific deficits in her profile of subtest scores on the WISC-R. Scholastic attainment testing showed that Sophie's reading, spelling and arithmetic skills were only marginally below her grade placement in the fourth grade at school, and these indices of achievement were within normal limits for her age. She was substantially younger than most of her classmates and was attending a school where the standards of achievement were higher than average, and these considerations had certainly contributed to the impressions that her parents had about here scholastic progress. Remedial action included counselling Sophie's parents and her teachers regarding their expectations of Sophie's educational potential and arranging for a period of additional tuition for the child, to consolidate basic literacy and number skills.

The treatment chosen for Sophie's bedwetting was the standard bed-pad and alarm conditioning procedure, combined with the waking schedule from the Dry-Bed Training procedure. The waking schedule was included because it was anticipated that this procedure would help to overcome Sophie's tendency to sleep deeply. The first step was to reassure Sophie and her parents that bedwetting is a fairly common problem, even for nine-year-olds, and that in her case it represented nothing more than a mild habit deficiency that was probably linked to her mother's childhood bed-wetting. It was stressed that the problem was not serious and that, if she followed the treatment procedures recommended, the prospects for a complete recovery would be high. The rationale underlying the treatment of her bedwetting was carefully explained, as described in Chapter 2.

For a period of two weeks prior to the commencement of treatment, Sophie was required to record each bedwetting incident as it occurred on a chart which we provided, and this recording confirmed that she was wetting every night. Following this time, which in effect established the baseline against which the effects of treatment could subsequently be compared, the practical requirements of the full procedure were described in detail, with the aid of a mock-up bed and the role-playing requirements as outlined in section 2.3. Sophie was encouraged to take responsibility for the procedure but, because of her age, it was anticipated that her parents would need to give her some assistance, at least during the initial stages of treatment. Written instructions were issued for future reference about procedural details, together with forms for record-keeping, these forms being set out as a calendar. Sophie's calendar was effectively a star chart on which she was asked to place a reward sticker for each dry night, (see Figure 2.4, p. 61). Her parents were required to keep a more comprehensive record, including details of Sophie's bedtime, the time of night when the alarm was triggered, any episodes of self-awakening for toileting, the size of the wet patch, when dry nights occurred and other information relevant to the child's progress such as illness, noncompliance with instructions, or equipment malfunction (see Figure 2.3 p. 60).

After treatment had begun, Sophie was required to contact the therapist once a week by telephone at a specific time, so

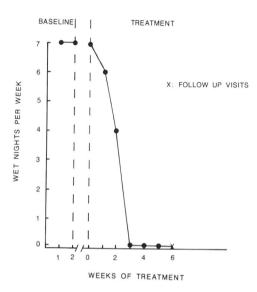

SOPHIE: aged 9 years

Figure 3.1 Record of Sophie's treatment

as to report on her progress. The parents were encouraged to make contact immediately if difficulties arose before the designated contact time. A follow-up interview was arranged with Sophie and her parents four weeks after the commencement of treatment.

It was agreed that the dryness criterion would be 28 consecutive dry nights. Use of the alarm was to continue until Sophie had achieved 14 consecutive dry nights and when this criterion was met she was to remove the apparatus from her bed but was to keep it at home until she had achieved a further 14 consecutive dry nights. Treatment ceased and the apparatus was returned to the therapist when Sophie had been dry for 28 consecutive nights. Before treatment began, the parents promised Sophie that they would reward her with a new quilt for her bed when she had achieved this dryness criterion.

Sophie's progress during treatment is summarized in Figure 3.1. She was dry during the first night of training, presumably because of the hourly awakenings, but then wet the bed on each of the six subsequent nights. During the second week of treatment she recorded four wet nights but thereafter she did not wet the bed again, recording 28 dry nights in a row and therefore meeting the success criterion. Follow-up at three months, six months and twelve months revealed that she had maintained nocturnal continence, with no relapses whatsoever.

A significant side-effect of the treatment in this case was the clear improvement in Sophie's general behaviour which accompanied the treatment. Both her parents and her school-teacher reported that Sophie had appeared to gain further confidence and self-assurance while following the enuresis programme. Her social life had become more active because, as she confirmed, she felt more confident about sleeping overnight at friends' houses and having friends stay with her.

3.2 Treating a diurnal and nocturnal enuretic child

Rebecca was aged six years at the time of referral. She had an eight-year-old brother and a three-year-old sister. She lived in a rural area and her parents were running a medium-sized farm in partnership with the father's two brothers and Rebecca's paternal grandfather.

The history described by the parents was that they had begun Rebecca's toilet training in the summer following her second birthday. However, she had not appeared to understand what was required and they had therefore abandoned her training until the summer of the following year. On the second occasion, Rebecca had mastered bowel control but had continued regular wetting during both the day and the night. She had been beginning to display some improvement in her bladder control at the time when her baby sister was born but this event appeared to set her back and frequent enuretic incidents resumed.

Enuresis continued unabated throughout her year in kindergarten and her first year at school and at about this time her parents became sufficiently anxious about the problem to seek professional help. Until now, they had attempted reward systems, lifting during the night for toileting, fluid restriction at bedtime and a twelve-month trial on imipramine. The drug treatment seemed to upset Rebecca's moods, however, and in addition was not effective in arresting her enuresis.

As we have commonly found, the initial interview uncovered some evidence of a family history of enuresis. Neither parent had experienced the problem themselves but the father had experienced past problems with urinary tract infections and described himself as having a 'weak bladder'. In addition, two maternal aunts and the maternal grandmother were reported to have been bedwetters during childhood. Both parents found it reassuring to learn that there is some tendency for bedwetting to occur within families but that the problem is usually readily overcome.

At the time of the initial interview, Rebecca's parents reported that she was having wetting accidents on virtually every day and night. Part of her problem seemed to reflect low functional bladder capacity, in that she appeared to receive little warning of the need to go to the toilet and she also voided more frequently than did her siblings. In view of the difficulties involved in precisely defining age-appropriate norms for functional bladder capacity, this was not actually measured in Rebecca's case but was assumed, using the observations made of the child's toileting habits. Moreover, a low functional bladder capacity did not provide a complete explanation and some behavioural element also appeared to be involved. Thus, the parents had noted that when engrossed in play, Rebecca would often show signs of needing to go to the toilet, like squirming while sitting down, clutching herself, and crossing her legs, but she would not respond appropriately until prompted by her parents. At school she often needed to go to the toilet during class because she found it difficult to hold on until recess and lunch breaks. However, she was frequently too embarrassed to ask the teacher in front of the class for permission to visit the toilet and, as a consequence, she had been having wetting accidents at school. Inevitably, these incidents attracted some teasing from other children and this appeared to be compounding the problem.

At the interview Rebecca was observed to be an extremely pleasant but passive and reticent child. By her own account, she managed her school work well and liked her teacher, but she had few friends at school. Furthermore, living on a farm in a fairly remote area, she came into contact with only a few children outside of school. Much of her leisure time was spent in play alone or watching television. In response to questioning about her enuresis she admitted to being bothered by this and she gave every sign of being highly motivated to pursue treatment.

It also became apparent during the initial interview that there were other family issues at hand that might have impinged on Rebecca's enuresis and that would need to be addressed as part of the treatment programme. A sibling of Rebecca's had died during infancy and the mother had suffered several miscarriages in the course of producing three healthy children. Moreover, the partnership arrangement for the family's farm was proving stressful for Rebecca's parents. This partnership was dominated by Rebecca's paternal grandfather and the father, who was an unassertive man, felt unable to cope effectively with this situation. Essentially, the father felt that he and his brothers were still being treated like children by their father and that, from a financial stand point, they were being manipulated. Thus, both of Rebecca's parents had experienced a great deal of emotional strain over the preceding years and much of this stress was still ongoing. The parents felt that their marriage was strong but admitted to being anxious and depressed and, indeed, they had each received medical help for these problems in the past.

Based on the assumption that Rebecca had a low functional bladder capacity, it was decided to start her on a combination of retention control training, together with treatment by the standard bed-pad and alarm programme, as described in Chapter 2. In respect of the retention control training, additional emphasis was placed on prompting Rebecca to use the toilet whenever she showed signs of needing to void but was delaying going to the toilet because of the distraction of play. It was also clear that Rebecca and her parents would need more counselling than usual and arrangements were therefore made to provide this. Follow-up sessions were to be longer than normal (up to 1½ hours instead of the usual 30 to 40 minutes). Though the parents lived in the country, they were prepared to visit the clinic in the city weekly during the initial phase of therapy. The schoolteacher was contacted by the therapist and an arrangement agreed to whereby Rebecca could leave the classroom unobtrusively without requesting permission whenever she felt the need to go to the toilet. The teacher agreed to keep a closer eye on Rebecca during class and in the playground, in order to remind her to go to the toilet if this appeared to be necessary.

Counselling of the parents centred on issues such as helping them to develop more assertiveness, particularly within the extended family, encouraging them to clarify their legal position in respect of the farm ownership and finances associated with their work, and breaking out of their social isolation. It was apparent that all members of the family as a whole needed to develop their social skills.

Rebecca's progress following treatment is summarized in Figure 3.2. It may be seen that her bedwetting frequency decreased rapidly during the first week of training but then seemed to flatten out, with reduced regular bedwetting incidents over the ensuing seven weeks. The frequency of her bedwetting then increased, this change coinciding with a particularly stressful period for the family, during which time the father confronted the paternal grandfather about his right to autonomy in his share of the farm management. Finally, there was a sharp improvement in Rebecca's bedwetting frequency and, after 16 weeks of treatment, she reached the dryness criterion, which in her case was 21 consecutive dry nights.

The improvement in the diurnal enuresis followed the same pattern as her bedwetting though, in general terms, this was less dramatic. At the end of 16 weeks of nocturnal treatment she had not completely stopped wetting during the day but the frequency had been reduced to approximately two

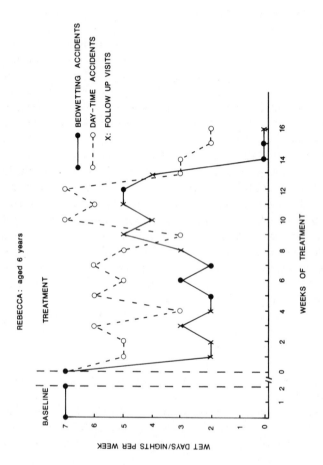

Figure 3.2 Record of Rebecca's treatment.

wetting accidents per week and these were described as being no more than tiny damp patches on her pants. Rebecca and her parents felt able to cope with this, without the need for regular follow-up.

At a follow-up six months later the mother reported that Rebecca still needed prompting to go to the toilet but, that, with this attention, she had remained dry during both the day and night. She had had only a very small number of isolated wetting accidents during the preceding six months. The mother also reported that Rebecca had recently received a very positive school report and that the child was looking forward to her promotion into the second year of primary education. Her parents had been attempting to develop Rebecca's social skills by inviting other children around to play and by encouraging her to participate in a school vacation swimming programme. Finally, the parents had formed a company in order to lease their share of the family's property with a view to purchasing the land two years later. Overall, Rebecca's mother felt that family relationships were now far less tense. Thus, Rebecca's case appeared to be one where identifiable stressful situations within the family were associated with the child's enuresis. Addressing those situations appropriately did seem to advance the success of behavioural treatment.

3.3 A case of intractable bedwetting

Occasionally one encounters an enuretic child who does not respond to the urine-alarm procedure in spite of high motivation and diligent effort on the parts of the child, the parents and the therapist. In this category was a boy whom we shall call Tom. He was referred at eight years and eight months with a lifelong history of bedwetting. His frequency of bedwetting at the time of referral was reported to be highly variable but during a two-week baseline period it averaged out at three to four wet nights per week. He had not experienced any difficulty with diurnal bladder or bowel control. His mother had been a bedwetter herself as a child but there appeared to be no other family history of enuresis. In response to specific questioning about depth of sleep, the mother said that she felt that Tom had no unusual sleep characteristics. During the initial assessment it was also revealed that Tom had a number of allergies which necessitated a special diet that was free from dairy foods. He suffered from moderately severe asthma, for which he was on a daily regimen of medication, and he also had severe eczema covering about 50% of his body. In spite of all these troubles, Tom had borne up remarkably well. He was a quiet but extremely pleasant and co-operative child and he enjoyed school, where he had many friends and coped well academically. Tom had had numerous medical examinations over the years for his various complaints. Urine analysis had revealed trace protein but this phenomenon was only evident when he was standing and it was considered by the referring paediatrician to be of no significance in respect to Tom's bedwetting.

The family lived in a country town where the father was a train driver and the mother did part-time cleaning work. Tom had an older brother and a younger sister, neither of whom had had any significant medical or psychological problems. The parents considered the various relationships within the family to be very healthy. Both parents were closely involved in the activities of their children and they had the backup of support from grandparents and an extended family in their home town.

Given this background, Tom was started on the standard bed-pad and alarm programme, with very high expectations for success. The programme was essentially the same as that already described for the preceding case studies in terms of alarm usage, record keeping and follow-up. His progress is summarized in Figure 3.3. From the outset Tom woke rapidly in response to the alarm, he took full responsibility for cleaning up after all bedwetting episodes and he kept his record diligently. It will be seen from Figure 3.3 that the frequency of his bedwetting reduced over the treatment period but his symptoms were never completely arrested. Although his longest dry period was 25 consecutive nights, beginning towards the end of the 21st week, the dryness

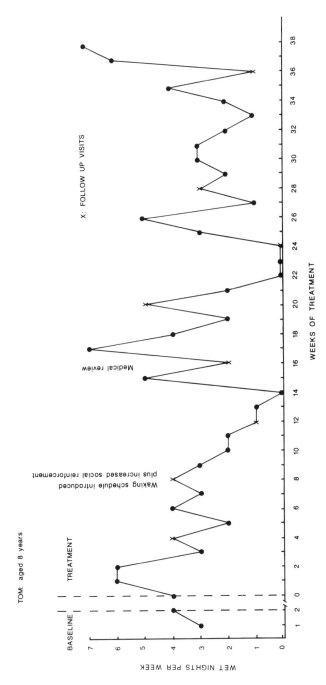

Figure 3.3 Record of Tom's treatment.

criterion agreed upon beforehand in his case had been 28 consecutive nights, because of his variable baseline bed-wetting pattern. Treatment continued for 38 weeks and towards the end of this time it was apparent that he had begun to slip back. One of the interesting features of his performance throughout, however, was that the diameter of the wet patch very rarely exceeded 2–3 inches (5–8 cm).

Various strategies were added to the bed-pad and alarm procedure in the course of treatment in an attempt to effect a complete cure. The waking schedule from the Dry-Bed Training procedure was introduced after two months, not because of difficulties when arousing Tom from sleep since he was already waking readily in response to the alarm, but in order to increase his chances of experiencing a dry night as a result of emptying his bladder during the night and thereby bolstering his confidence.

Steps were taken to increase the amount of social rein-forcement that Tom received, by encouraging his grand-parents, with whom he was very close, to take an active interest in his progress. Further, other family members and close friends were asked to praise him regularly whenever he managed to have a dry night. Specific targets were established with Tom to encourage him to attempt to reduce weekly bedwetting incidents gradually during treatment. A system of rewards was introduced for achieving these short-term, more immediate improvements in performance, but culminating in a new bicycle if he was able to become fully continent. He was also given the retention control exercises from the Dry-Bed Training procedure, as described in section 2.4. There was a distinct improvement in his response after the introduction of these additional procedures but not enough for him to achieve complete continence.

After the programme had been going for four months, Tom was again reviewed medically but still no underlying physical abnormality was found. Eventually, after 38 weeks without him reaching complete continence, his treatment was terminated. Tom was told that, while he had tried very hard, the programme was not working and it would be best to have a break and to resume the treatment at some later time.

Persisting with the urine-alarm programme for 38 weeks prior to discontinuing is longer than normal but this had been done in Tom's case because he was so determined and had wished to continue.

It is difficult to know why the programme failed to arrest Tom's bedwetting, although in retrospect we could see that there were several possibilities. Firstly, the consistently small patch that was formed as a result of his bedwetting incidents could have been the consequence of a form of dribbling incontinence and this raises the possibility of some uncommon form of organic pathology not detected by the medical review. Cases like Tom may warrant more extensive investigation than the mandatory physical examination, micro-urine analysis and blood pressure check that Tom received. However, the parents were not keen to pursue further medical investigations because these can be quite unpleasant and Tom had already undergone many demanding medical procedures as a consequence of his asthma. The parents therefore preferred to wait and see whether the bedwetting would be resolved without further intervention, for example as a result of maturation, or if it would respond to a second trial with the bed-pad and alarm at a later date. This situation has remained unchanged throughout a twelve-month follow-up period; Tom still continues to wet the bed regularly but, in view of his many other problems, his parents have regarded his bedwetting as a relatively low treatment priority.

A second possible explanation for the failure of Tom's programme is that since he was such an allergic child it is possible that his enuresis was associated with some form of allergic reaction. We also considered the possibility that a common denominator for Tom's various illnesses might have been a high level of anxiety, sufficient to interfere with conditioning, but this seemed unlikely in our opinion because Tom has not shown any overt signs of anxiety during our contact, either at home or at school. In our opinion, the most likely explanation for Tom's poor response is bound up with the medication he was taking for asthma. One of the drugs which he was taking was theophylline, which is known to affect smooth muscles, of the kind that are present in the bladder. This drug is also a diuretic and therefore results in an increased production of urine. Certainly, in our experience there appears to be a disproportionate number of asthmatic children on similar medications who also wet the bed and who are particularly difficult to train using the bed-pad and alarm device.

3.4 A case of prolonged low-frequency bedwetting

Daniel was a little over nine years old at the time that he and his parents agreed to seek treatment for his bedwetting. According to his mother, who made the initial approach to the clinic, he had always wet the bed but the pattern of wetting was reportedly erratic, varying from one or two wets in a week to four or five. His mother could not recall for how long this pattern had been maintained but was certain that Daniel had never been dry and believed that the pattern of low frequency wetting dated from late infancy – perhaps from about four or five years of age. Daniel was the third child among four, having two older brothers and a younger sister. The other three had all been enuretic and the girl (aged seven years) was still wetting the bed at the time that Daniel commenced treatment. The two older brothers had spontaneously become dry between about seven and eight years of age.

It was Daniel's persistent bedwetting beyond this age, coupled with his own embarrassment and desire to be rid of the problem, which had finally persuaded the mother to seek help. Hitherto, her attitude had always been markedly permissive; by the parents' own account Daniel's father had long considered that outside intervention was warranted but the mother had consistently resisted this, insisting that the bedwetting was not important and that Daniel would become dry in his own time. This permissive attitude towards bed-wetting appeared to be characteristic of general child-rearing practices within the family. The father, a senior public servant, seemed easygoing, kind and gentle, and happy to view the responsibility of raising the children as his wife's province. Her personality appeared to be very similar to his and all of her interests seemed to be focused within the home, principally on her children. From the outset, prior to when treatment actually began, she insisted that treatment would only proceed because Daniel wanted it to and that, should he change his mind, treatment would cease immediately.

The first meeting with Daniel and his parents established that apart from the bedwetting, Daniel's development in every other regard was completely satisfactory. Although IQ was not measured, he was clearly an intelligent child and his school reports confirmed that his progress at school had always been excellent. At our request, Daniel's mother arranged for him to undergo a thorough medical examination prior to commencing treatment but this found no evidence of any physical immaturity or any organic abnormality. Daniel, in short, had an average build for his age and seemed both physically and psychologically well-adjusted in every way, apart from the poor nocturnal bladder control. There was some evidence of a family history of bedwetting, not only involving Daniel's siblings but also including a cousin of Daniel's, related on his mother's side. However, neither parent could remember whether either they or others in their families had encountered problems as children in acquiring nocturnal dryness.

Daniel's treatment formed part of a research project which we were conducting into the efficacy of Dry-Bed Training when this was carried out by the parents at home. Following the mother's initial contact with the clinic, we visited Daniel and both his parents at their house, so as to discuss what would be required and especially to go through the full Dry-Bed Training procedure with them, including the bed-pad and alarm equipment, retention control training, positive practice, and the waking schedule, as already described in Chapter 2. Next, Daniel established a baseline for wetting, against which any subsequent improvement associated with treatment could be evaluated. He recorded each bedwetting incident as it occurred for four weeks, thereby establishing that, as his parents had claimed, the extent of his bedwetting was not stable, but varied between two and five wet nights a week.

From the outset, Daniel and his parents assumed the full responsibility for his treatment. We visited the house again on the afternoon before treatment began, in order to check the arrangements made and to go over all aspects of the procedure with the parents once more. A telephone call next morning confirmed that the first night of intensive training had passed smoothly, without any procedural difficulties, and a home visit one week later found the family well-adjusted to the treatment regimen. At this meeting it was agreed that a weekly telephone call by the therapist to the mother should suffice to collect Daniel's record of bedwetting episodes. The mother also agreed that she would keep an independent record, so as to provide an indication of Daniel's reliability when maintaining his own chart.

Thereafter Daniel's progress was rapid, as may be seen from Figure 3.4. He had only one wetting episode in the next week and by the end of the fourth week of treatment he had already achieved 14 consecutive dry nights. As part of the programme, the bed-pad had been removed from Daniel's bed after the first seven dry nights. The parents reported that on one occasion during the first week of this fortnight they had forgotten to check that the alarm was set, after arriving home late after an evening out, and that it was turned off when they checked the following morning. However, Daniel had not in any case wet the bed on that night, so that no harm was done. However, two days later Daniel's mother contacted the clinic, in a state of some concern; Daniel had wet the bed after 15 dry nights in a row and had wet again on the following night. He was reportedly excessively upset by these events and did not wish to continue with the programme of treatment. She was also reluctant to persevere, realizing that under the procedure being followed she would have to reintroduce the waking schedule for the next several nights, and the cleanliness training routine following any further wetting accidents.

As a consequence, the therapist visited the family at home that evening and, after considerable discussion, Daniel was

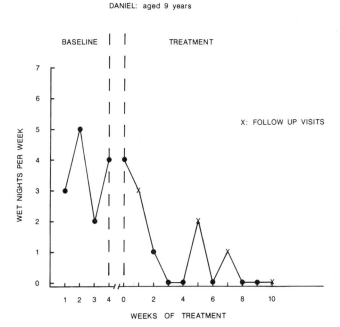

Figure 3.4 Record of Daniel's treatment.

persuaded to try again, it being pointed out to him that he had already come close to a cure and that he had little to lose and everything to gain from continuing. Treatment resumed that night and no further accidents occurred for the remainder of that week, throughout the next week, or for the first six nights of the week following (the seventh week of treatment). However, on the last night of that week, after 17 dry nights in a row, Daniel wet the bed once again.

The effect of this accident was nothing short of traumatic, triggering a day-long tantrum by Daniel which was so severe that he had to miss school that day. By the time the therapist had responded to the mother's telephone call by visiting the house mid-morning, the whole family was involved, including not only the other three children but both pairs of grandparents as well. At first Daniel seemed literally inconsolable and the mother was adamant that treatment must cease forthwith. None the less, at least one other adult, the maternal grandmother, seemed convinced that Daniel should persevere and, sensing an ally in that quarter, the therapist set to work to see if Daniel and his parents might be persuaded to go on. In the event they were persuaded and Daniel never wet the bed again. He finally achieved the dryness criterion of 21 consecutive dry nights at the end of the tenth week and registered no relapse at follow-ups twelve months and two years after the termination of treatment.

3.5 Treating a child who does not wake readily to the alarm

Joshua was nine years of age at the time of referral. He was referred initially by an ear, nose and throat surgeon, for an assessment of school-related problems. The background to these problems was a long history of recurrent ear infections throughout infancy and early childhood, with associated intermittent hearing loss. However, for a period of two years prior to our contact, Joshua's general health had been excellent and recent comprehensive medical investigations had revealed that he had not suffered any permanent impairment to his hearing. None the less he continued to have difficulties at school, reports from his teachers noting inconsistent work. Teachers also noted that Joshua's concentration in class was poor and that he appeared to have problems with short-term memory. However, there was a general feeling among his teachers that he was capable of better grades, although in terms of his general manner and behaviour at school he had always attracted very favourable comments.

At the first meeting at the clinic the therapist formed the opinion that Joshua was a really delightful lad. He was relaxed and chatty and generally seemed to be a pleasant, well-adjusted boy. He completed the Wechsler Intelligence Scale for Children (WISC-R), which established that his level of general intelligence was within normal limits and an examination of his basic literacy skills revealed only minor lags in reading, spelling and arithmetic. Further tests were conducted in light of the school reports about his poor concentration and short-term memory and, indeed, these tests confirmed that his performance in these areas was below the norms for children his age. In view of his normal IQ it seemed unlikely that Joshua had a significant learning disability, although his school achievement was generally below what might be expected given his IQ. It was therefore decided, that with the co-operation of his class teacher, to introduce a remedial programme at his school, to focus on developing his listening and short-term memory skills.

In the course of this contact, it was learned that Joshua was also a bedwetter. The relevant background to this problem was that he had acquired day-time urinary control by about two years of age. He was much slower to acquire bowel control and, indeed, had continued to experience occasional soiling accidents during his first two years at school. He had never acquired nocturnal bladder control, and at the time of the initial assessment he was wetting the bed several times during each night. The family history suggested the possibility of some inherited component, in that both parents had been bedwetters themselves as children. The mother had been treated with a bed-pad and alarm device, which had successfully arrested her symptoms when she was about five years of age. The father, on the other hand, had outgrown the problem by about seven years of age, without the need for special treatment. Certainly, the parents' perception of Joshua's bedwetting was that he had inherited the problem from them. In addition, they were adamant that he was an exceptionally deep sleeper.

Joshua's parents had been very active in treating his bedwetting in the past. In light of the mother's experience as a child, they had placed most faith in the urine-alarm procedure but three separate trials with an alarm, one extending over eight months, had failed to arrest his symptoms. On each occasion Joshua seemed to have great difficulty in rousing in response to the alarm. The third of these treatments had actually been the full Dry-Bed Training programme, and it is of particular interest that during this programme Joshua's difficulties at school had become most acute. On reflection, the parents felt that this programme had made Joshua anxious and frustrated and that it had had a generally detrimental effect on his behaviour. It is worthwhile noting too that, in the opinion of the parents, these three trials with an alarm had not been adequately supervised. Two had involved equipment hired from a local pharmacy which had provided written instructions only. The Dry-Bed Training programme had been organized by a local community health centre but, apart from an initial interview, no follow-up instructions had been provided. Joshua's parents had also tried to treat his bedwetting with medication (imipramine), which had almost immediately lowered the frequency of his bedwetting, but the level of bedwetting had then seemed to reach a plateau. Furthermore, as soon as the medication had ceased, Joshua's bedwetting frequency had slipped back to at least once every night.

On the occasion reported here it was decided to reimplement the bed-pad and alarm procedure, combined with the waking schedule from Dry-Bed Training, and other strategies aimed at facilitating waking in response to the alarm. Essentially, these additional strategies were, first, the use of an alarm that emitted a very loud and complex signal, rather like a burglar alarm. Secondly, if Joshua did not respond to the alarm after a minute or so, one of his parents was to attend to him, using physical prompts, ranging from a gentle shaking to placing a wet cloth on his face, in order to rouse him. Thirdly, the parent was then required to accompany him through the rest of the procedure of toileting, remaking the bed and resetting the alarm, so as to ensure that these procedures were done properly.

Joshua's progress is summarized in Figure 3.5. It can be seen that although the numbers of bedwetting episodes were substantially reduced, particularly during the initial weeks of treatment, his progress appeared to stall and he continued to wet regularly, though less frequently, without reaching the dryness criterion. Thus, when progress was reviewed after 12 weeks of treatment, the parents reported that Joshua was still not responding reliably to the alarm. Furthermore, they were aware that on several occasions he must have turned the

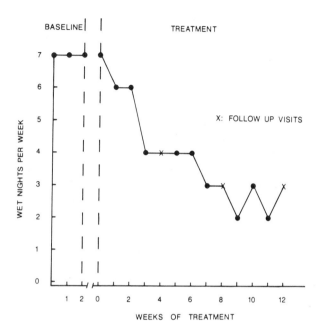

Figure 3.5 Joshua's first treatment.

alarm off and returned to bed, without going through the other required procedures of toileting, remaking the bed and resetting the alarm, since his bed was wet the next morning and the alarm had been set properly the night before. The parents felt that Joshua was doing this virtually 'in his sleep' because he had no recollection of the event next morning and because at other times he appeared to be very highly motivated to become continent. These incidents established that the parents themselves often did not hear the alarm and therefore were not able to assist Joshua in the manner planned. In part, this may have been because the two bedrooms were not adjacent and the parents considered that they themselves were both deep sleepers.

At this point the mother raised the possibility of Joshua being helped by way of hypnosis, which she suggested might at the very least sensitize him to the sound of the alarm. Consequently the therapist contacted a medical practitioner who specialized in hypnotherapy and who was very confident about being able to arrest Joshua's bedwetting, without the need for using any alarm device. Joshua attended six weekly sessions of hypnotherapy and at the end of this period the hypnotherapist wrote back to the therapist, claiming that Joshua's bedwetting symptoms had now been arrested as predicted. However, a few weeks later the parents contacted the therapist again with the disappointing news that Joshua had resumed wetting the bed with high frequency. They reported that during the course of hypnotherapy Joshua's bedwetting frequency had been reduced to about two wet nights per week but then had not improved beyond this; this was the criterion that the hypnotherapist had used to discharge Joshua from treatment.

Joshua and his parents were by this time extremely doubtful about the likelihood of him becoming dry. None the less, he and his parents were prepared to persist with treatment using the bed-pad and alarm device, providing an arrangement could be made to overcome the difficulties associated with his failure to awaken following bedwetting accidents. Accordingly, arrangements were made for a second treatment to begin. The alarm procedure described above was used again but on this occasion an extension speaker was also placed in the parents' bedroom. Under this arrangement the alarm was triggered simultaneously in the bedrooms of Joshua and his parents, thereby enabling the parents to awaken more reliably and to attend to Joshua.

It can be seen from Figure 3.6 that under this new treatment regimen Joshua's progress was again relatively slow but steady and on this occasion he was successful in obtaining the very stringent dryness criterion of 28 consecutive dry nights. At follow-up after 12 months he had maintained nocturnal continence.

The problem of children failing to arouse to the alarm is fairly common and parents often need reassurance about this. In fact, many children are slow to respond to the alarm early on in treatment although most gradually become more

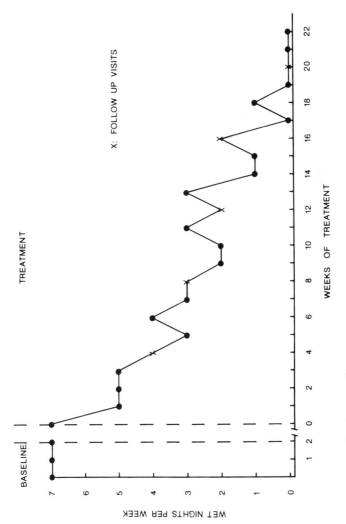

Figure 3.6 Joshua's second treatment.

responsive as treatment proceeds. However, when failure to awaken persists beyond the initial stages of treatment, and it is clear to the therapist that no motivational problem is involved, then the procedure which we introduced with Joshua on the second occasion is one which is worthwhile trying.

It might be noted at this point that we have actually sometimes treated some enuretic children successfully, without them ever waking in response to bedwetting events. Presumably, in these cases the effect of the alarm has acted directly on the bladder sphincter and achieved the same desired response. Such cases are fairly rare, however, and as a general rule children who awaken readily to the alarm do show the best overall response to this form of treatment.

3.6 Treating persistent relapse

Gavin was aged seven years at the time of referral. He had the common history of having wet the bed on virtually every night of his life and, indeed, his parents had established that on most nights he was wetting more than once. They had been lifting him during the night for toileting and, when doing so, had frequently found that he was wet at the time of being lifted and that, further, his bed was wet again on the following morning, after he had been awoken. Gavin had always displayed excessive frequency and urgency of micturition during the day and had been slow to acquire diurnal bladder control. At the time of the initial interview, he was still experiencing occasional day-time wetting accidents. The parents remarked that it was quite usual for Gavin to be engrossed in play but then suddenly to make a last minute dash to the toilet, only to begin voiding on the way. His parents had also noted that, in addition to voiding more frequently than their other children when they were at the same age, the volume of urine passed by Gavin at each voiding was relatively small. Moreover, Gavin's urinary stream seemed to be weaker; it consisted of a short stream followed by a prolonged period of dribbling and he often had slightly damp pants as a result of this residual dribbling.

A medical examination prior to the initial psychological assessment, including micro-urine analysis and a blood pressure check, failed to reveal any underlying physical abnormality. At the assessment interview, Gavin gave the impression of being an intellectually bright, self-sufficient and socially competent child. It was established that at school he was in the top group of his class, he was average to good at sport, and he had many friends. He was able to talk openly about his bedwetting, stating that his parents had never criticized him for the problem, and nor had he attracted teasing from his siblings or from people outside of the family. None the less, he had recently become extremely frustrated by the continual wet beds and he was highly motivated to be rid of the problem.

The family appeared to be a close-knit one. Both parents were school-teachers, with the mother now working on a part-time basis only, and there were no obvious financial pressures or other domestic strains of significance. Gavin was the youngest of four children. His parents placed high emphasis on academic achievement, though none of the children appeared to be pushed beyond his/her capabilities. The parents were very sympathetic towards Gavin's difficulty, partly because the mother had been a bedwetter as a child until about ten years of age. None the less, they had attempted a variety of remedial strategies with Gavin, including fluid restrictions and reward systems, in addition to the night-time toileting arrangement mentioned above, but all without success.

Gavin was treated using the standard bed-pad and alarm programme, in conjunction with the waking schedule from Dry-Bed Training. In light of the overall presentation of the problem, expectations for success were high. Weekly telephone contact times were arranged to monitor his progress and personal meetings once a month were also planned, these to continue until the dryness criterion of 21 consecutive dry nights had been reached.

Gavin's progress is shown in Figure 3.7. It can be seen that he made slow but steady progress and eventually reached the dryness criterion after 25 weeks of treatment. At this point

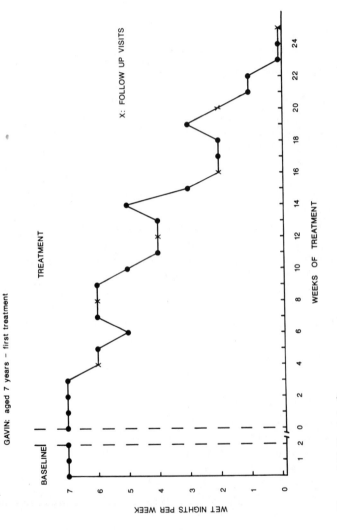

Figure 3.7 Gavin's first treatment.

Gavin and his parents met with the therapist in order to return the equipment and to enable the therapist to reward Gavin for his achievement. In addition, as has already been mentioned in Chapter 2, it is common practice to meet with children and their parents in this way in order to discuss the issue of possible relapse. Gavin was assured that, having achieved this period of dryness, the odds were that he would no longer be bothered by the bedwetting problem. However, it was acknowledged that there was a possibility of relapse and that this might involve a further trial with the alarm apparatus. It was suggested to his parents that if Gavin was to have an occasional wet bed in the future, the best policy would be to treat it as an unfortunate accident, but not to attach any more significance than that to any isolated bedwetting event. However, if subsequently bedwetting was to become more frequent and regular, like, for example, more than one wet bed per week over a period of one month, then the parents should contact the therapist immediately.

Approximately three months later Gavin's mother telephoned to report that Gavin had relapsed and was wetting the bed regularly again. This had begun with an isolated wet bed, but such incidents had then rapidly increased in frequency. The mother was advised to resume keeping a formal record of Gavin's bedwetting frequency and arrangements were made to reinstitute the bed-pad and alarm programme as quickly as possible. By the time that the second trial on the alarm had been started, Gavin was again wetting the bed every night. He was disappointed to have slipped back but nevertheless remained highly motivated and confident that his symptoms would be arrested on this occasion. The original treatment regimen of the alarm combined with the waking schedule from Dry-Bed Training was used again for this second trial.

Figure 3.8 summarizes Gavin's progress during the second period of treatment. It can be seen that his response was again slow, compared with the majority of enuretic children who undertake this programme, although the duration of the second treatment was somewhat briefer than the first. Gavin again reached the dryness criterion of 21 consecutive dry

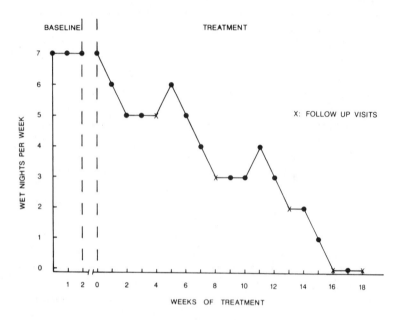

Figure 3.8 Gavin's second treatment.

nights and at this point the programme was stopped and he was given the original follow-up instructions regarding the possibility of further relapse.

Within the next four months Gavin relapsed again. On this occasion his mother contacted the therapist as soon as Gavin's bedwetting frequency had reached approximately two accidents a week on average. Arrangements were made for him to be reviewed medically and these investigations again revealed no underlying physical abnormality. However, his parents still regarded him as having a 'weak bladder', although by this time he was having very few wetting accidents during the day. None the less, his parents had noted that on long car trips Gavin would be the first member of the family to need a toilet stop and he generally appeared unable to hold on before voiding for as long as other children of his age. For this reason, it was decided at this time to add retention control training to the programme previously followed – that is, the bed-pad and alarm, together with the waking schedule.

Essentially, the retention control training given to Gavin was the same as the procedure described in section 2.4. That is, each afternoon after arriving home from school Gavin was required to void in the toilet. He was then given a large drink and encouraged to hold on for as long as possible before emptying his bladder in the toilet. He was also encouraged to practice starting and stopping the urine stream when voiding. It was also decided that when Gavin had again reached the dryness criterion, then an additional overlearning procedure would be introduced, in an attempt to reduce the likelihood of subsequent relapse. Thus, after he had achieved 21 consecutive dry nights the programme was changed so that he was then encouraged to drink as much as he could, immediately prior to retiring to bed for the night.

Gavin's progress during the third period of treatment is summarized in Figure 3.9. By the commencement of treatment, his bedwetting frequency had crept up to approximately four accidents per week. His response to treatment on this occasion was quicker than previously and he reached the dryness criterion within approximately ten weeks from the commencement of training. At this point the overlearning procedure was introduced as planned and subsequently he wet his bed on three occasions during the next five weeks. However, when the overlearning procedure was discontinued, he maintained dry beds for the next three consecutive weeks and at this point all treatment procedures were stopped.

Gavin maintained dry beds for approximately six months before the by now familiar pattern reappeared, with isolated accidents quickly developing into regular bedwetting. By this time Gavin was approximately ten years of age and he had been involved with the treatment for his bedwetting in one form or another for almost three years. He and his parents were becoming extremely frustrated and starting to despair that he would ever be rid of the problem. None the less, they were prepared to persist with treatment.

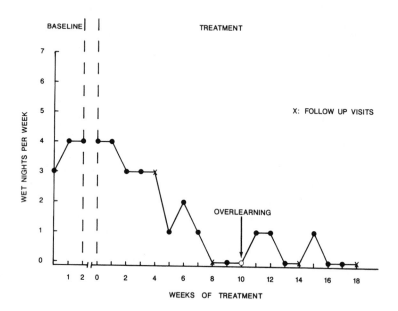

Figure 3.9 Gavin's third treatment.

For the fourth treatment programme it was decided to employ an intermittent reinforcement schedule, since this is a commonly used variation on the standard bed-pad and alarm procedure which is aimed at reducing the likelihood of relapse. Thus, a programme was devised whereby the bed-pad and alarm system was to be set to sound on a variable ratio basis, in response to approximately 70% of Gavin's bedwetting accidents, estimated from the frequency of bedwetting during the baseline period. This meant that the alarm was set to ring, on average, on three nights in seven. Retention control training during the day was stopped since his parents had not noticed any increase in his functional bladder capacity while using these exercises. The waking schedule was also dropped, since by this time Gavin awoke reliably and very rapidly in response to the alarm. Since he was wetting only twice per week at the commencement of the

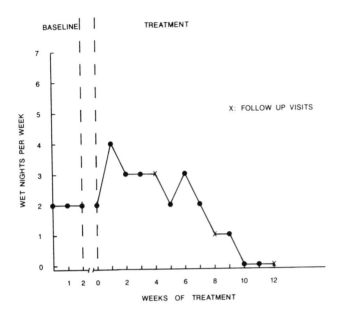

Figure 3.10 Gavin's fourth treatment.

fourth treatment trial, it was decided to retain the overlearning procedure and Gavin was encouraged to increase his fluid
intake immediately prior to bedtime. He understood that this
should increase the likely number of wetting accidents but
that these would provide increased subsequent opportunities
for reinforcement by way of the alarm. Gavin's progress
during the fourth period of treatment is summarized in
Figure 3.10. Once again his symptoms were arrested, this
time within approximately ten weeks, and after 21
consecutive dry nights the programme ceased.

Over the next three years, Gavin continued to experience
further relapses in his bedwetting. By this time Gavin and his
parents had become reconciled to the possibility that he may
require several ongoing periods of treatment with the alarm
before permanent bladder control would be achieved. In the
end they purchased their own bed-pad and alarm equipment,

which they used without direct therapist supervision as soon as it had become apparent that Gavin had relapsed again. Altogether, they used the alarm, without any adjuvant procedures, on about five further occasions before Gavin finally achieved permanent nocturnal continence.

In retrospect, it can be seen that there were some definite trends in Gavin's response to treatment. Initially, his symptoms were slow to arrest but his response during the second and third treatments became increasingly more rapid. He was somewhat slower to respond on the fourth occasion, during the period of intermittent reinforcement, but this is a tendency that has been commonly noted when this form of therapy has been used. Thus, intermittent reinforcement schedules, while lowering the likelihood of relapse in some cases, generally take longer to arrest bedwetting symptoms in the first instance. Furthermore, there was a trend towards each subsequent relapse being less severe than the previous one. In other words, at the beginning of treatment Gavin was wetting the bed several times each night but each subsequent relapse involved a progressively lower wetting frequency.

It is difficult to account for Gavin's persistent relapses. As mentioned earlier, he impressed as being an intelligent and highly motivated boy and there was never any doubt about his full compliance with the treatment programme. In retrospect, it seems plausible that Gavin was a case where slow physiological maturation played a significant role in proneness to relapse. It is also difficult to know whether any of the additional procedures used to supplement the standard bed-pad and alarm programme (i.e. retention control training, the waking schedule, intermittent reinforcement, overlearning) helped at all. Clearly, if there was any benefit from these procedures it must have been minimal because Gavin continued to relapse over a lengthy period of several years.

While approximately 40% of children treated with the bed-pad and alarm device do relapse after achieving initial dryness, the incidence of multiple relapses, as occurred in Gavin's case, is fortunately very small. One of the lessons learned from the treatment of Gavin is that a valid approach to adopt when multiple relapses appear might be simply to view treatment as a very long-term process that will involve a series of 'booster' trials using the bed-pad and alarm until permanent dryness is achieved. Certainly, Gavin and his parents were able to reconcile themselves to this position after their initial disappointment. In such cases, acceptance of the need for several trials on the alarm may be aided by the knowledge that successive treatments are generally shorter in duration and that the periods of dryness between relapses generally become longer and longer. Gavin's case also underlines the value of warning parents, when describing the procedure in the first instance, of the possibility that their child may well require more than one trial on the alarm before permanent remission is achieved.

3.7 Treating a noncompliant child

David was a most reluctant participant when bought along by his mother for the initial assessment interview. He was a good looking, well-developed twelve-year-old but he was very sullen and detached throughout the interview. Communication was dominated by the mother who openly expressed her annoyance and frustration with David's bedwetting in front of him. David's mother reported that he had wet the bed regularly all of his life, in spite of being toilet trained for day-time bladder and bowel control by about two years of age. Over the past few years he had been seen by various professional people with regard to the bedwetting problem, including four separate referrals to an enuresis clinic at a large public hospital. These periods of treatment in the enuresis clinic had involved use of the bed-pad and alarm procedure for a total period of about 18 months but these treatments had not been successful in arresting his symptoms. Other forms of treatment had included medication (imipramine), which the mother reported had made him emotionally labile, so that treatment was discontinued after a few weeks. Hypnotherapy had also been tried but David thought that this was 'stupid' and he had refused to attend after the initial two sessions. A combination of fluid restriction and a waking schedule had also been attempted but his parents had found these difficult to implement, largely because of David's noncompliance. However, an interesting feature of David's history was that a few years earlier the family had holidayed overseas and during this period of three months David had been completely dry at night. His longest dry period at night apart from this time overseas had been about seven days. He had never shown particular concern about his bedwetting even though he was now approaching adolescence.

His school reports had consistently noted that David had a high intellectual potential but that he had achieved only mediocre results because of a poor attitude towards study. The school reports commented in addition on his unwillingness to socialize with other students and his reluctance to participate in sport, even though he was a physically strong and well-coordinated boy. His mother also expressed her concern about David's school performance, asserting that this was consistent with poor behaviour and attitude at home as well. All of this information was passed on by the mother in front of David in a highly critical, angry tone – to which he displayed a smug attitude of seeming indifference.

It was readily apparent from the initial assessment interview that the primary reason for David's lack of success with previous treatments had been his poor compliance with the procedures to be followed. This noncompliance appeared to be associated with a general attitudinal/motivational problem on his part that was in turn related to relationships within the family. In particular, there appeared to be a great deal of animosity between David and his mother. None the less, there did not appear to be immediate prospects for dealing with these difficulties and it was decided to attempt the bed-pad and alarm programme again but under conditions of closer than normal therapist supervision in order to combat the compliance problem. It was arranged that David should come to the therapist's office each week so that progress could be reviewed. David was required to take full responsibility for the programme, including washing his soiled bedding, and for the record-keeping. The parents were

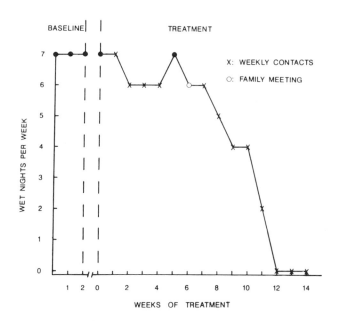

DAVID: aged 12 years

BASELINE   TREATMENT

X: WEEKLY CONTACTS
O: FAMILY MEETING

WET NIGHTS PER WEEK

WEEKS OF TREATMENT

Figure 3.11 Record of David's treatment.

encouraged to be as supportive and positive of David's efforts as possible, but otherwise to leave the responsibility of monitoring his progress to the therapist. This approach was particularly emphasized to the mother.

As can be seen from Figure 3.11, David's baseline bed-wetting frequency was seven wet nights per week. He showed only some slight improvement during the initial few weeks of treatment and during this time, too, he made excuses for late or non-attendance at weekly meetings and his record keeping became sloppy. After six weeks of treatment the therapist met with both parents and David and it was revealed that after the first few weeks David had not been using the alarm as instructed (he was simply not switching it on at night) nor was he bothering to change his bedding following bedwetting accidents. The mother kept her part of the bargain by resisting from nagging David but it was quite clear that she was extremely frustrated and that she was struggling to control her feelings.

At this point, the family dynamics were explored in more detail. David's father was an intelligent man in his mid-forties who was a clerk employed in a government agency. He was not ambitious, his position involving only a moderate degree of responsibility, and he viewed work merely as a means of earning sufficient income to make ends meet. He liked to be able to come home after work, have his evening meal and relax in front of the television. David's mother, on the other hand, was much more dynamic and volatile. She also worked, as a nurse's aide, on permanent night shift. Thus, during the week the parents were rarely at home together. The mother was well-organized, having meals prepared in advance and always keeping the house tidy. However, she was frustrated by untidiness on the part of the other family members. She frequently complained that she would leave for work with the house tidy, only to return to find all her work undone and no-one else appearing to care, and she would explode in response to this. Other family members perceived her as attempting to run the family like a 'boot camp' and would frequently respond by becoming even more lax. The mother also made it quite plain that she did not respect her husband's lack of ambition and failure to contribute to a more healthy, outgoing family lifestyle. David had an older sister at university who seemed to cope with the family quarrels by spending as little time at home as possible.

These issues were discussed by the therapist and both parents in some detail and the option of more formal family therapy was put to them but was declined. They did, however, agree to try to observe some basic ground rules which could minimize the effect of family quarrelling on the treatment of David's bedwetting. Essentially, it was agreed that the father would take more responsibility for ensuring that David used the bed-pad and alarm as required and that he followed through his responsibilities to clean up, keep accurate records and attend weekly appointments with the therapist. For the mother's part, it was re-emphasized that she should try to refrain from finding fault with her husband

and other members of the family – something which she thought she might find easier to do once the father became more active in David's management. The other significant modification to the programme was to require David to telephone the therapist daily so as to report on his progress, in addition to the weekly personal visits. A specific time for telephoning, prior to setting off for school, was arranged.

These modifications appeared to improve David's compliance and his progress thereafter was much more pleasing. It will be seen from Figure 3.11 that, following the family meeting and the instigation of the above modifications, David improved steadily. He reached the dryness criterion of 21 consecutive dry nights after a further eight weeks of treatment using the alarm. At the time when treatment was discontinued, the quarrels and differences within the family were far from resolved and it was anticipated that David would probably relapse to regular bedwetting. However, follow-up over the next twelve months revealed that he experienced only sporadic wetting accidents and no major relapse.

Essentially, this case demonstrates that very close therapist supervision is an effective means of dealing with children who do not satisfactorily comply with treatment procedures. There may be other effective strategies as well; in this particular instance, family therapy aimed at resolving the entrenched and complex difficulties involving communication between the various family members might have been effective but this form of intervention was not acceptable to the family members themselves.

Another possible strategy for dealing with noncompliant children is the use of the positive practice procedure taken from Dry-Bed Training (i.e. the requirement that the child counts to 50, goes to the toilet after every bedwetting episode, and repeats this procedure 20 times before returning to bed). However, this is a very demanding procedure for both the child and parents to implement and, in the authors' experience, it can produce markedly different outcomes, depending on circumstances. Thus, it may have the effect of either a dramatic breakthrough in achieving compliance, or the opposite effect of actually increasing noncompliant behaviour. For this reason, positive practice is probably most useful for speeding up the progress of children who are, in fact, already highly motivated and complying with treatment procedures to begin with.

3.8 Treatment involving a noncompliant family

Neil was eleven years old when he was referred to the enuresis clinic of a large metropolitan hospital. The initial interview with him and his mother revealed that Neil had been somewhat later than normal to acquire initial bladder and bowel control during the day. However, this control had been firmly established by the time that he was about three and a half years of age. At this time also he had begun to achieve nocturnal bladder control and, indeed, he had been reliably dry at night for a period of several months. Subsequently, bedwetting incidents gradually reappeared and, though the frequency was variable at the time of our initial contact, he was averaging three to four wet nights per week.

Neil's bedwetting had attracted a great deal of attention and concern from within the family. He was the youngest of six children, all of whom were still living at home. He had two older teenage brothers who were still attending school and three older sisters who were attending university. Neil's father had completed a bachelor's degree at university and now managed his own sharebroking business, which was not a large concern but which was thriving and demanded at lot of his time and energy. None the less, the father still attempted to play an active role in family life. The mother had also had a university education but she was now engaged full-time with home duties and it was clear from our discussions that she had been more involved than the father in the child-rearing process.

There was no family history of enuresis and the other members of the family found it difficult to understand Neil's problem. Reactions ranged from sympathy, mainly from his mother and his sisters, to annoyance on the part of his father and derision from his brothers. The mother had initiated referral for treatment because of a growing awareness that Neil was becoming acutely embarrassed and anxious about his bedwetting. Over a period of time she had observed a steady deterioration in his self-confidence, social involvement and school performance. In addition, while Neil took full responsibility for cleaning up after bedwetting accidents, the mother was frustrated by the continual demand to wash extra sheets and to air out the bedroom.

In spite of the parents' concern about Neil's bedwetting, relatively little had been done in the past to deal with it, mainly because of the father's firm belief that Neil should be able to conquer the problem himself. Neil had had a trial on medication (imipramine) which had helped a little but this method of treatment had in any case been discontinued after a few weeks because of the father's ambivalence about the use of medications with children. About the only behavioural strategy that they had employed regularly was the practice of lifting Neil at night for toileting. The mother was of the opinion that, if it were not for the fact the Neil had been woken during the night for toileting, his bedwetting frequency would have been virtually every night. During the initial assessment interview at the clinic the mother also noted that Neil was a very deep sleeper.

At that interview, Neil impressed as a bright, alert and very sensitive lad. He was in the top academic stream at school, where he achieved good average grades without having to extend himself too far. He was not a dominant figure at school but he was popular with the teachers and other students. He was highly embarrassed and reluctant to talk about his bedwetting and a good deal of reassurance and encouragement from the therapist was required before he would open up and talk about the problem. He stressed that he had tried very hard to avoid wetting the bed but that, for some reason which he did not understand, he was unable to remain dry consistently. Once relaxed, Neil went on to say that he was ridiculed by his brothers about his bedwetting. Neil and his parents had taken elaborate precautions to keep the problem within the family but often his brothers would threaten to tell everyone at school. Further, Neil related that while his parents did not overtly say or do anything unpleasant regarding his bedwetting, he sensed his father's disappointment in him and his mother's concern and frustration.

Establishment of a baseline wetting frequency (i.e. without Neil's mother lifting him during the night for toileting) confirmed the mother's belief that without this help Neil was wetting the bed every night. Following the baseline period, the standard bed-pad and alarm procedure, combined with the waking schedule from Dry-Bed Training, was implemented. The essential difference between Neil's case and the other cases reported here was that a greater emphasis was placed on the psychological preparation of Neil. Thus, he was strongly reassured about the prevalence of bedwetting, even among children of his own age, and that if he persisted with the programme as described, then the prospect of arresting his bedwetting would be very high. In addition, the therapist discussed ways with him by which Neil could deal with his brothers' possible reactions to the introduction of the programme. The mother, who was the only parent who attended the initial interview, was given similar reassurances. In particular, it was pointed out that the programme should not necessitate extra work for her, since Neil was prepared to take full responsibility for his bedwetting episodes; and the requirement to wake him nightly according to the waking schedule would only be formalizing a practice that she had already been employing for many years.

Neil's progress during treatment is summarized in Figure 3.12. At the first follow-up interview, Neil and his mother showed only mild enthusiasm about his progress, since the overall bedwetting frequency achieved during the first three weeks of treatment had remained high and was essentially no different to what had previously been achieved by waking him without the adjunct of the alarm. None the less, his record showed that the size of the wet patch had decreased significantly over the four-week period and both Neil and his mother were also encouraged by the fact that he had not wet on four consecutive nights immediately prior to our meeting.

Neil improved dramatically during the next four weeks

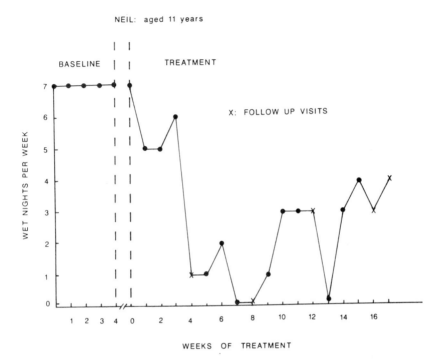

Figure 3.12 Record of Neil's treatment.

and, indeed, at the time of our next meeting he had been completely dry for 16 consecutive nights. However, it was apparent from the record that he had been waking himself, in addition to any scheduled waking by the mother, in order to maintain dry beds. Further questioning revealed that Neil's brothers had complained about the disturbance of the alarm and had generally made him uncomfortable about his participation in the programme. One brother, with whom Neil shared a bedroom, had sometimes switched off the alarm after Neil had gone to bed in order to prevent himself being awakened by Neil's bedwetting. Thus, Neil was more frightened than ever about wetting the bed. However, while he had developed the ability to wake himself during the night, and thereby maintain dry beds, this seemed to interfere with his normal sleep pattern, to such an extent that he was beginning to show signs of fatigue and lethargy during the day.

The family's support for the treatment programme was reviewed with the mother. She was aware of the brothers' intolerance towards Neil's participation but felt unable to do much about this attitude. The arrangement of the house did not allow for Neil to have a room of his own. She felt that the sisters had been quite supportive of Neil but confirmed that the father had remained sceptical from the outset. None the less, Neil and his mother were now delighted with his achieving so many dry nights, so that, in spite of the difficulties described, they decided to persevere with the programme until Neil had attained the prearranged dryness criterion of 21 consecutive dry nights. It was also apparent that Neil at this point was not confident enough to return the alarm.

At the third follow-up visit it was clear that there had been a general deterioration in Neil's progress. The number of wet nights had increased significantly and, associated with this, Neil's confidence and compliance had suffered. He tearfully related that his brothers had become extremely annoyed about being disturbed by the alarm and that, as a result, he had not been turning the alarm on each night before retiring. In addition, he felt very disappointed that he had been unable to attain the dryness criterion of 21 nights, after getting so close.

Attempts were made to arrest the increase in the frequency of Neil's bedwetting, firstly by providing him with supportive counselling. Extra support and encouragement was sought from other family members and the sisters proved most responsive in this regard. The father had become more sceptical than ever, however, any by this time the mother herself was beginning to have serious doubts about the likely success of treatment. The therapist also requested an interview with the brothers to review their role in Neil's treatment. One brother attended and gave some indication that he was prepared to become more supportive. However, the other brother refused to attend the appointment and, if anything, elevated the amount of criticism that he had already been directing towards Neil and the enuresis programme.

At the next and final visit it was obvious that Neil had reached a stalemate. Effectively, he had not been using the alarm at all, his bedwetting frequency had increased to the pretreatment level, consistent with his mother lifting him during the night, and his confidence was badly eroded. By this time both parents had become completely cynical about the programme and, all things considered, it was proving to be anti-theraputic. Thus, the equipment was returned, it was suggested that all pressure and attention to Neil's bedwetting be stopped, and that the situation be reviewed in six months time. Predictably enough, the review appointment was not kept and a follow-up telephone conversation with the mother revealed that Neil's bedwetting frequency was back up at the pretreatment level.

In hindsight, there were several factors that contributed to Neil's failure to respond to the programme but those that stand out are the father's negative attitude towards the treatment from the outset, the brothers' sabotage of the programme, Neil's absolute disappointment at getting so close to the dryness criterion only to wet again and, ultimately, Neil's noncompliance with the treatment routine. It is possible that this situation might have been managed better had the therapist been more assertive with the father and the brothers. The father and one of the brothers did not have any personal contact with the therapist throughout the time that the treatment programme was running. Perhaps a family therapy approach, in conjunction with the alarm procedure, or at least an initial meeting in the child's home with all the family members present would have been more effective. In view of the pressure that Neil was under and his fragile confidence, more frequent contact between Neil and the therapist than the monthly meeting, interspersed with occasional telephone calls, may well have been beneficial also.

3.9 Treating an adolescent

Angela was 14 years of age when she was referred to a hospital enuresis clinic for treatment of her bedwetting. An assessment interview established that Angela had been toilet trained initially without difficulty for bladder and bowel control by about two and a half years of age. However, she had continued to wet the bed from that time and subsequently had never really established nocturnal bladder control, although she had experienced some periods of dryness. As a younger child she had wet the bed on virtually every night and, while this frequency had decreased with age, at the time of referral she was still wetting two to three nights per week on average. The longest period for which she had remained continuously dry that she could recall was about three months.

Furthermore, in the past Angela had experienced difficulties with urinary frequency and urgency during the day. This had led to occasional wetting accidents at school while she was in her early grades, and to consequent teasing by other students. Although the day-time accidents had ceased to occur by the time that she had reached third grade at about seven years of age, this experience seemed to some extent to have impaired her social interaction. Indeed, she had had a stormy passage through primary school in the area of peer group relationships. At the time of referral she was in year 10 at secondary school where she was coping well academically. Socially, she was out of the mainstream, though not entirely isolated, having managed to establish a small circle of close friends.

Angela's family situation was noteworthy for at least two reasons. First, there was a history of enuresis within the family; an eight-year-old sister had had a bedwetting problem and still wet the bed sporadically, and Angela's father, though defensive about this matter, apparently had also wet the bed as a child. Secondly, there had been significant emotional upheaval within the family, resulting from the parents' separation and divorce five years earlier. Angela's bedwetting was well established prior to this, but her parents' separation and the associated emotional *sequelae* were disturbing for Angela, particularly because it appeared to her that her parents' separation had occurred without warning. There were six children in the family and, following the separation, Angela, along with three of her siblings, lived with her mother. One sibling now resided with her father and another had moved in with the maternal grandmother. As far as Angela's situation was concerned, her mother had experienced considerable financial hardship associated with her having to bring up four children on a government pension for a single supporting parent and a great deal of tension was associated with Angela having access to the noncustodial father and to her siblings who lived away from the maternal home.

The initial contact between the therapist and Angela got off to a bad start. Firstly, the letter confirming an appointment had been sent to her father's address, the change of address in her medical notes not having been noted following the separation. As a consequence, Angela was angry and embarrassed that her father knew of her contact with the enuresis clinic. Also, there had been a last-minute postponement of her first appointment at the clinic. Thus, at the time of the initial interview she impressed as a very attractive and athletic teenager who was bright intellectually and who had quite sophisticated communication skills; but she was also prickly and negative, appearing to over-react to questioning about her circumstances and to take offence where none was intended. Thus, while her anger and distrust could be attributed in part to the unfortunate blunders associated with the appointment, it did also seem to reflect a tendency towards general moodiness, and her school reports consistently contained teachers' comments to this effect.

Considerable time was necessary to establish the beginnings of an adequate communication with Angela but eventually she felt able to confirm that her bedwetting was the major source of most of her frustration and worry, but she also admitted that she was confused in her feelings about her parents. She went on to say that she had already attempted many treatment procedures in the past, including a trial with a bed-pad and alarm device, but nothing had seemed to help. She saw the present contact as a final effort to get rid of the problem.

Much of this initial discussion focused on reasons why previous treatment with a bed-pad and alarm device had not resulted in dryness. Previously, she had hired an unreliable system from a local pharmacy and she and her mother had been left to administer the procedure on their own, without any supervision or back-up. In discussion, however, she seemed reassured that a further trial with a bed-pad and alarm would be the best treatment to pursue. It was pointed out that this would have a higher likelihood of success than her previous experience with an alarm, because this time it would involve more sophisticated equipment and closer supervision. Furthermore, she was promised that, in light of her overall circumstances, closer involvement than usual with the therapist would be available.

Angela had made it known during the assessment interview that there were many things about school and home that she would like to discuss with someone at some later time but that she needed more time to build up an appropriate amount of trust in the therapist. Arrangements were therefore made to see her on a weekly basis at the clinic after school, for half hourly sessions which combined supportive counselling with the usual monitoring of progress in the bedwetting programme. Finally, it was suggested that she should take full responsibility for the programme at home. It was possible for her to move to a room on her own for the duration of the treatment and her mother agreed that virtually all of the follow-up should be between Angela and the therapist.

Angela's progress was highly variable during the initial stages of treatment. There were difficulties in establishing rapport between Angela and the male therapist. On occasions during the follow-up sessions she would comment that there were things that she wanted to talk about with someone but that she felt too embarrassed to discuss them with him. Her bedwetting frequency, which is summarized in Figure 3.13, did not really alter during the initial weeks

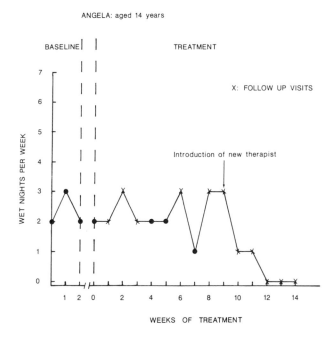

Figure 3.13 Record of Angela's treatment.

of treatment and Angela expressed disappointment at first about the lack of improvement. Subsequently this disappointment was converted into anger which was then directed against the therapist. Essentially her attitude was that the treatment had failed in the past, that the present therapist had promised that it would work this time – but that it had not. In all, she felt let down; her attendance at follow-up meetings became irregular and her compliance with the alarm procedure became erratic. After eight weeks, the overall situation was reviewed with Angela. She quite bravely asserted to the therapist that she found it difficult to relate to him and she requested a female therapist. This was arranged immediately, so that a programme of weekly counselling sessions, in conjunction with the bed-pad alarm procedure, continued along with no major break in the treatment, apart from the lapses in compliance that had already occurred.

Following the change to a female therapist for all follow-up sessions, Angela's progress improved rapidly. She reached the dryness criterion of 21 consecutive dry nights within six weeks of transferring to the new therapist. Follow-up appointments at three, six and twelve month intervals revealed that she had maintained her nocturnal continence and her mother, who attended these follow-up appointments, reported an improvement in Angela's social and emotional adjustment. In general terms she appeared to be a much happier and more settled person.

Subsequent discussion between the two therapists involved with treating Angela revealed that she had had some quite phobic feelings about aspects of her enuresis. In particular, she feared that the bedwetting would never be resolved and that this would stifle relationships with boys and ultimately inhibit the development of normal sexual relationships. She also found it very unpleasant when her bedwetting occurred during her menstrual cycle. In addition, she had for a long time harboured a deep seated fear that the enuresis represented some form of sinister physical and/or emotional disorder. However, she had not felt able to discuss such feelings with a male therapist, particularly those relating to sexual relationships and to the management of bedwetting during her menstrual cycles.

On reflection, there are several lessons to be learned from this case about the management of teenage bedwetters. Firstly, there may be a higher likelihood of emotional factors being bound up in the problem and these will require attention if progress is to be made. We have already discussed a possible association between emotional disturbance and enuresis, holding the view that, for the vast majority of children, emotional problems are likely to be the result of continuous bedwetting rather than the cause of it. Even in

Angela's case this was probably so although, clearly, there were other significant stresses in her life, particularly the family upheaval associated with her parents' separation and divorce. However, it still appeared that the embarrassment and inconvenience of wetting the bed as a teenager was the major source of Angela's anxiety and in her case this anxiety did appear to interfere with initial attempts to treat the enuresis. Thus, whatever the source of her anxiety, the emotional reaction had to be dealt with in therapy. This required alternative arrangements at the clinic and more therapist contact, a situation that has proved subsequently to be not atypical when treating adolescents, who we have found often require a greater emphasis on supportive counselling than is usually necessary with younger bedwetters. Secondly, as with any theraputic intervention, one is reminded of the need to establish appropriate rapport between the therapist and patient from the outset. In this case there appeared to be specific reasons for choosing a female therapist. Thirdly, the impact of previous attempts at treatment is more relevant with teenagers because they are older and have had more opportunity for past treatment. Thus, the reasons for any previous failures need to be dealt with and, particularly if a bed-pad and alarm device has been tried before, then suitable reassurances must be provided about why this method is expected to be effective on the present occasion. In a similar vein, any myths associated with the teenagers' thoughts about the origin and nature of the bedwetting problem and its ultimate prognosis will need to be dealt with. Finally, in this and other cases involving teenagers, it is desirable to allow the teenage enuretic to take full responsibility for the programme. While parents certainly have an active supportive role, most of the contact time in therapy is usually between the therapist and teenager.

3.10 Treating a defiant adolescent

Amanda was 15 years old when she first came for psychological assessment and advice. As was the situation with Sophie in the first case study, bedwetting was not the primary reason for referral and Amanda was described by her parents as having an 'attitude problem', both at home and at school. Thus, she was said to be very casual in her approach towards study and the performance of routine domestic chores. She was not engaged in any organized sporting or extra-curricular activity but, instead, spent much of her time watching television or listening to music. In addition, her parents considered that she was too young to be going out to parties and dances but she was becoming very interested in these activities and quarrelled with her parents as a consequence. In fact, her parents' disallowance of these activities had led Amanda to sneak out late at night on weekends to meet with her friends. She was prickly in her attitude towards her parents and her younger siblings and in general terms she was defiant of basic family rules. These behavioural characteristics had apparently always been present to some extent but had become more intense since Amanda reached adolescence. Her defiance was also becoming increasingly apparent in her behaviour at school as well as at home. Whereas in earlier grades she had been a good student, her scholastic performance had now declined and she was reported to have become a disruption in class. She was frequently testing the authority of her teachers, being cheeky and generally being rebellious.

In respect of her enuresis, Amanda had been effectively toilet trained for day-time bladder and bowel control before the age of 2 years. She had been rather slow to establish nocturnal bladder control but this appeared to have been achieved by about 4 years of age. She remained continent at night (with only very occasional accidents) for the next 6 years or so. Thereafter she began to wet the bed sporadically. Thus, she was capable of dry periods at night for 6 months or more, but these were followed by periods of frequent bedwetting lasting for several months. On reflection the parents felt that there was an association between the onset and severity of Amanda's bedwetting and other pressures in her life. The problem was thought to be most severe, for example, around examination time at school or when things had been particularly stressful at home. With the deterioration in Amanda's behaviour during the two or three years prior to our contact, and the consequent elevation in family tensions, Amanda's bedwetting at the time of referral was worse than ever, occurring virtually every night. The parents had not sought formal help for the problem previously, apart from occasional chats with the family's medical practitioner who was a long-term family friend, because they preferred to keep the problem to themselves. The local doctor had also checked Amamda periodically from the medical point of view and the possibility of underlying organic pathology had already been excluded. The parents were unaware of any strong family history of enuresis although the father conceded that he may have wet the bed himself up until school age. The parents had not noticed anything unusual about Amanda's pattern of sleep.

Family relationships in this case were particularly relevant. Amanda was the eldest of three children, her sisters being aged ten and eight years. The father was a senior partner in an international firm of management consultants and the mother was a solicitor working in private practice, with a large, well-established law firm. The mother had been out of the workforce when her children were younger, but when the last of the children was settled at school some three to four years prior to our contact, she returned to work full-time. Both parents prided themselves as being 'self-made'. In other words, they each had come from humble family origins, they had progressed through the government school system and they both had achieved their respective positions through hard work. They were heavily involved with their occupations which demanded long hours each day, and the father in particular was frequently away from home on business. While the parents' achievements were admirable, their attitudes and values did appear to be somewhat self righteous and less tolerant of others. Their work ethic was clearly evident in their attitude towards their children, who were expected to excel at virtually everything that they attempted. Mediocrity, and/or laziness, were scorned. Amanda, being the eldest, attracted most pressure from her parents to perform well. She also had the additional pressure of supervising her younger sisters in the after-school hours, prior to her parents' return from work.

In interview, Amanda impressed as a physically attractive and mature adolescent. She was very defensive to begin with and it appeared that she viewed the therapist as another authorative figure to be treated sceptically. Thus, considerable effort was required initially to establish rapport by talking with Amanda on her own before even broaching the topic of enuresis. Once a climate of trust had been established, however, Amanda was able to express her anger and upset about the way in which her parents related to her. She felt that they expected more from her academically than she was capable of achieving and she felt burdened by the responsibility of having to look after her sisters after school, an activity which had the effect of curbing any normal after-school activities that she might otherwise have shared with her peers. She felt particularly irritated by the parents' constant reminders that she enjoyed the benefit of attending a private school and all the material advantages that the parents themselves had lacked as children. She recalled feeling guilty as a younger child when the parents made these comments but now she reacted with defiance. She regarded her parents' comments as nothing more than nagging and she disregarded them accordingly. Moreover, she was aware that her bedwetting was something that greatly annoyed her parents and while she reported not consciously wetting the bed and being keen to be rid of the problem for her own sake, she admitted to receiving some satisfaction for being able to 'get back' at her parents by way of her bedwetting. She also admitted to engaging in other behaviours, like avoiding homework and sneaking out at night, for the same reasons.

Early intervention with Amanda involved a standard psychometric assessment, since poor scholastic performance was part of the presenting problem, and also because there was some uncertainty on the part of the therapist about

Amanda's actual abilities. Results from WISC-R suggested that her abilities were solidly within the average range, indicating that she had the potential to cope adequately but without being outstanding at her stage of secondary schooling. Furthermore, test results suggested that she would have to work very diligently to manage study at a tertiary level, which, however, her parents had automatically presumed she would pursue. Significantly, prior to discussion about the outcome of the assessment with Amanda, her father telephoned the therapist and insisted that under no circumstances was the therapist to communicate to Amanda that she was incapable of managing university studies. Consequently, the implications of the assessment in respect of Amanda's scholastic performance and behaviour were discussed with the parents and a compromise was reached, in which the parents agreed to be more supportive and positive in their management of Amanda who, in turn, agreed to be more compliant. It was accepted that Amanda was capable of somewhat better performance at school with reasonable effort but that she was unlikely to ever become a top-stream student. The possibility of her progressing to university was not ruled out but it was suggested that in the course of her final secondary school year she and her parents should consider alternative tertiary courses and career paths, in the event that Amanda did not gain entry into university.

Having done this groundwork, attention was focused on treatment of Amanda's enuresis, using the standard conditioning programme. In light of her age and the particular family dynamics it was suggested that Amanda should take full responsibility for the programme, including toileting after wetting episodes, re-making the bed, record keeping and reporting to the therapist. Figure 3.14 shows her progress.

It can be seen that at the beginning of treatment Amanda was wetting the bed six to seven nights per week on average. She improved significantly during the first few weeks of treatment but thereafter slipped back to her baseline wetting frequency. At the follow-up interview after

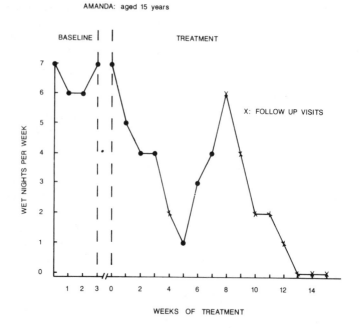

Figure 3.14 Record of Amanda's treatment.

eight weeks of treatment it was learned that there had been renewed clashes between Amanda and her parents over her school performance. As a result, Amanda had become lax in her compliance with the enuresis programme. Thus, she was not consistently following the prescribed procedures for setting the alarm, emptying her bladder in the toilet following bedwetting episodes, and changing the soiled bedding, and her record keeping had become very careless and inaccurate. Her mother had been particularly aggravated by several episodes in which Amanda had dumped the wet sheets on the bedroom floor instead of depositing them in the laundry. When left in the bedroom for a day or more the soiled sheets had resulted in an unpleasant smell that had spread through the house. Following these episodes the mother had felt unable to maintain a passive role in the treatment programme and had begun waking Amanda when the alarm was triggered and supervising all of the required treatment procedures. Amanda resented this, so that she and her mother were in dispute, with neither party willing to concede ground.

Further counselling followed, again emphasizing the desirability of Amanda taking full responsibility for the bedwetting programme, without direct parental involvement. In addition, weekly follow-up visits with the therapist were arranged. During these follow-up sessions the benefits to Amanda of achieving continence were discussed with her, in a way which separated these from what she perceived to be her parents' wishes. With this closer supervision and supportive counselling, Amanda was able to achieve the dryness criterion of 21 consecutive dry nights. She remained dry for a further four months but thereafter relapsed, in effect replicating her past history of sporadic periods of bedwetting interspersed with quite long periods of continence. Amanda and her mother subsequently attended a review appointment. This made it clear that the regression in Amanda's bedwetting had again been associated with stormy outbursts at home, this time in response to her mediocre examination results. At this point it was recommended that the parents and Amanda should together seek family therapy prior to a further trial with the bedwetting alarm. Unfortunately, however, this approach was totally unacceptable to the father and neither family therapy nor the bed-alarm programme was pursued. Instead the parents decided to seek the help of their family doctor for a trial with imipramine. Thereafter, direct contact with Amanda lapsed. Her long-term outcome is unknown, although it is quite likely that medication would have helped to reduce the frequency of her bedwetting. We believe, however, that a complete cure would not be likely until Amanda left home and/or the conflicts between her and her parents were resolved.

3.11 Treating an intellectually disabled child

There have been relatively few studies into the treatment of bedwetting with intellectually disabled children, and most of these studies have involved institutionalized populations. None the less, the available evidence suggests that the urine-alarm procedure is effective in arresting bedwetting in intellectually disabled people, although success rates tend to be lower and the duration of treatment longer than is usually found among nondisabled populations.

Susan was 14 years of age when she was referred for the treatment of life-long bedwetting. A recent psychometric assessment using the WISC-R, showed her to have a full scale IQ of 46. Her intellectual disability was associated with hydrocephalus which had been present from birth. In addition, she suffered from epilepsy, which was well controlled by anticonvulsant medication, and from mild spasticity. She had been educated within a special school system where emphasis had been placed on the development of self-help skills and on the learning of activities for daily living. She was able to manage her day-time toileting requirements but she had always been a regular bedwetter. To this time no significant effort had been put into treating her bedwetting, presumably because it had been considered to be a direct consequence of her general intellectual limitations. Susan had also exhibited a number of major behaviour problems in the past although these had settled down to some extent with the passage of time. However, she was still easily upset and was prone to aggressive outbursts whenever she felt frustrated.

Bedwetting treatment for Susan was carried out in essentially the same manner as has already been described for a number of preceding cases. She was given the urine-alarm programme in conjunction with the waking schedule. Susan and her mother met with the therapist in his office in the usual manner for the initial assessment interview and for a demonstration of the procedure, although extra care was taken to ensure that Susan fully understood what was expected of her. While it was arranged that she should take as much of the responsibility for maintaining the programme as possible, it was assumed that she would need more parental assistance than would normally be required for a nondisabled 14-year-old.

In discussion with Susan's mother, additional emphasis was also placed on positive reinforcement for dry nights. Susan kept the simple star chart normally used by younger children (Figure 2.4, p. 61) and here mother kept a more comprehensive record of her progress (similar to that shown in Figure 2.3, p. 60). In addition to these standard follow-up techniques, however, the family was encouraged to praise Susan generously whenever she achieved a dry night. This praise was repeated several times during the day and she was reminded of her achievement the following night before retiring to bed. She was also rewarded with her favourite meals, choice of clothing and choice of favourite television shows following each dry night. These rewards had previously been determined as having particular value for Susan. Apart from the normal requirements that she get out of bed and switch off the alarm, finish voiding in the toilet, dry the enuresis pad and remake the bed, there were no other aversive consequences as a result of a bedwetting episode.

Susan's progress is summarized in Figure 3.15. Initially she seemed highly motivated and she co-operated well with all aspects of the treatment programme. She was obviously delighted by the reward schedule and her early progress was good, with a significant reduction in bedwetting frequency being obvious within the first few weeks. Gradually, however, she became less co-operative and she began to sabotage the programme by switching off the alarm before going to sleep. This was countered by her mother, who normally retired later than Susan, switching the alarm back on after Susan had fallen asleep.

Over the ensuing weeks, although Susan maintained her improved nocturnal bladder control, she became increasingly frustrated and noncompliant. In response to this, some of the rewards were altered; e.g. she expressed an interest in specific social outings and these were therefore incorporated into the programme as rewards, contingent upon her achieving seven consecutive dry nights. After 36 weeks of perseverence, Susan achieved the dryness of four consecutive dry weeks. This is a stringent dryness criterion and was chosen because it had become apparent during training that

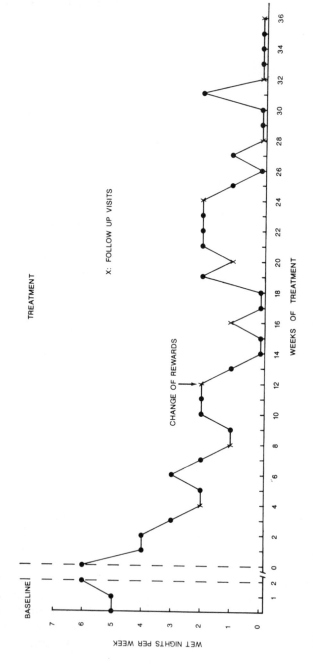

Figure 3.15 Susan's first treatment.

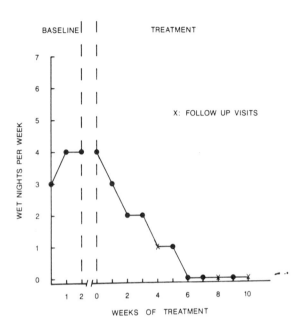

Figure 3.16 Susan's treatment following her first relapse.

she would commonly manage to be dry for a week or two but would then wet several times before again being dry for relatively long spells. This pattern of wetting during treatment has been reported by others working in this area with intellectually disabled children.

Susan maintained her nocturnal bladder control, with only occasional isolated accidents, for seven months. At that time her mother contacted the therapist to report that Susan was again wetting the bed with high frequency. However, the urine-alarm procedure and the waking schedule were immediately re-implemented and her bedwetting was arrested within six weeks, as shown in Figure 3.16. Her mother reported a second relapse four months later but Susan once again resumed treatment using the bed-pad and alarm, together with the waking schedule. As may be seen from

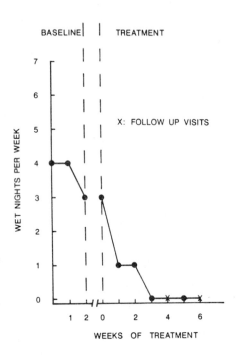

Figure 3.17 Susan's treatment following her second relapse.

Figure 3.17, on this occasion she wet the bed only twice before achieving the dryness criterion. She was subsequently followed up for 18 months but there were no further episodes of relapse.

3.12 Treating a child with associated emotional problems

Prue was seven years old when she was referred for psychological assessment and management by the family's general medical practitioner. Approximately nine months beforehand she had been involved in a motor vehicle accident in which she was a back seat passenger in the family's car being driven by her mother. After a collision with another car, Prue had been thrown forward and her head had become wedged between the two front seats. She had also suffered bruising to her thigh and groin and had sprained her ankle. She did not lose consciousness and had not suffered any significant head injury but she had been trapped between the front seats of the car for approximately 30 minutes before it had been possible to release her.

Prue's mother had been knocked unconscious as a result of the accident and she had also suffered very serious injuries to her knee and ankle which subsequently required orthopaedic surgery and which ultimately impaired her capacity to drive a car. Prue's teenage sister, the only other passenger in the car, had suffered a significant head injury involving loss of consciousness for several hours, and other injuries to her neck and ribs as a result of the buffeting. Prue had witnessed these very unpleasant injuries to her mother and sister in the immediate aftermath of the accident, during which time she had had her head wedged between the two front seats. Altogether it had been an extremely upsetting experience for her. Her physical injuries had been resolved without complication but, not surprisingly, she had shown signs of emotional disturbance and had exhibited a number of marked behavioural changes immediately following the accident. Initially she had insisted on sleeping with her parents but, even then, she had experienced nightmares almost every night. The nightmares had decreased in frequency by the time of our contact but she was still insisting on staying up until her mother retired to bed and she still insisted on sleeping in her parents' bed.

At the time of the first interview, Prue still exhibited an acute fear of travelling as a passenger in a car. At first she had simply refused to get into a car but this situation had improved to a point where she could travel as a passenger, although she was obviously tense and she now tended to be a back-seat driver. Her fears appeared to be exacerbated by her awareness that her mother's driving ability had been impaired by the injuries to her leg sustained in the accident. She had developed an acute separation anxiety immediately following the accident. Thus, she would panic when her mother was late to pick her up from school and she consistently sought information about her mother's daily movements. She was reluctant to play at other children's houses and, in general terms, seemed to have become more fearful, markedly socially withdrawn and noticeably unhappy. She also displayed a number of psychosomatic symptoms. In particular, she complained of vague aches and pains in her stomach and head and she also complained of blurred vision. These symptoms appeared to be impairing her scholastic performance. ·However, the symptom of most interest to the present discussion is that Prue had begun to wet the bed nightly, immediately following the motor vehicle accident. In addition, she had begun experiencing occasional day-time wetting.

All of the above symptoms contrasted with Prue's personality prior to the accident. Beforehand, she had been regarded as being a normal, happy and well-adjusted child. She had passed her developmental milestones briskly, she slept through the night undisturbed, she did not appear to be a nervous child and she certainly did not have any specific phobias. In addition, she had been completely toilet trained for both diurnal and nocturnal bladder and bowel control by about two years of age and she had maintained this continence, without any trouble, until the time of the accident. On the basis of this assessment, Prue was diagnosed as having suffered an acute post-traumatic stress reaction, as a direct result of the motor vehicle accident. Some of the major features of this reaction (separation anxiety, phobia for travelling in cars, sleep disturbance, psychogenic pain) had settled down somewhat with the passage of time but there were still significant emotional problems. Her secondary enuresis had shown no signs at all of abating.

The first step taken towards the treatment of Prue's bed-wetting was to attempt to reduced the intensity of her fears and her overall level of anxiety. This was put into effect using a combination of play therapy and systematic desensitization. Initially Prue and her mother met with the therapist for six one-hour sessions of therapy. The play therapy involved one-to-one contact between Prue and the

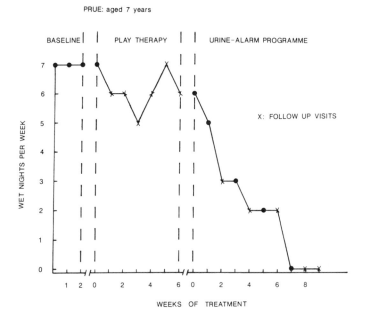

PRUE: aged 7 years

Figure 3.18 Record of Prue's treatment.

therapist, during which time Prue was encouraged to communicate her anxieties through the medium of play and other
activities such as drawing. The systematic desensitization
focused on reducing Prue's acquired dependence on her
mother, particularly with respect to her pattern of disturbed
sleep. This was dealt with by having the parents make up a
temporary bed for Prue next to their own bed. Thus, Prue
was required to sleep in the temporary bed, and as she
gained confidence, the physical distance between the
temporary bed and her parents' bed was gradually increased.
Eventually she was required to go down in her own bed at
a reasonable hour. If she woke during the night she was
allowed only a brief cuddle in her parents' bed and
reassurance from her parents, before having to return to her
own bed. As may be seen from Figure 3.18, these procedures
produced very little effect on the frequency with which Prue
wet the bed and, once she was able to sleep comfortably in

her own bed, the bed-pad and alarm procedure was implemented.

Prue's progress once treatment had begun is summarized in Figure 3.18. It can be seen that the frequency of Prue's bedwetting during the period of play therapy was less than the seven nights per week recorded by her parents during the initial baseline period. Presumably there had already been a slight improvement during the period of psychotherapy involving the combination of play therapy and systematic desensitization. In any case, once the bed-pad and alarm procedure had been introduced she improved dramatically, attaining the dryness criterion of 14 consecutive dry nights after only seven weeks of alarm usage. At a follow-up six months later it was reported that Prue had maintained her nocturnal continence. The other symptoms associated with the post-traumatic stress reaction had also improved but the parents were of the opinion that she was not yet fully recovered from all of the effects of the accident.

This case represents an example of secondary enuresis which follows acute emotional upheaval. In many cases, secondary nocturnal enuresis will be associated with emotional problems that become chronic in nature, such as a breakdown in family relationships, ongoing problems at school or difficulties with peer group relationships. In any event, it is likely that some form of psychotherapeutic input, combined with the bed-pad and alarm procedure, can be effective in arresting the child's bedwetting symptoms. Nevertheless, in some cases the onset of secondary nocturnal enuresis occurs for no apparent reason at all. In these instances, introducing the bed-pad and alarm procedure on its own is usually successful in arresting the bedwetting.

3.13 Treating a child with multiple disabilities

Mary was born to a mother who had had a known psychiatric illness since childhood. The mother had also contracted rubella during the early months of the pregnancy and Mary had been born with a severe hearing impairment. She also had cataracts and a heart defect, and weighed only 2 lbs 15 ozs (0.6 kg) at birth. The parents had been repulsed by their abnormal baby and had moved away from South Australia to another state, leaving Mary in hospital for three months before returning and taking her home. Unfortunately, the mother did not respond to the child who, as a consequence, suffered physical neglect and emotional deprivation until the age of 16 months, by which time she had malnutrition, could not sit up and simply lay in her cot staring at her fingers all day. At that time Mary was taken by her maternal grandmother for a six-week stay and her grandmother taught her to sit and to stand. However, she deteriorated quickly when she again returned to her parents, who separated a short time later.

At 21 months of age Mary was placed into the full-time care of her maternal grandparents. The situation then appeared to be stable until about twelve months later, when her grandfather died and her grandmother could no longer cope physically or financially with Mary. Subsequently Mary was made a ward of the state and went to live in a cottage home for deaf children, attending a special kindergarten for the deaf. Her care at weekends and holidays was shared by a number of different private homes and agencies. When about three years of age, Mary was referred to the Department of Psychiatry at a large metropolitan hospital where a psychological assessment estimated her intellectual functioning to be below that of an 18-month-old child. In addition, she was thought to be very disturbed emotionally and it was known that she was by now a significant management problem in the cottage home. A comprehensive behaviour modification programme was implemented within the cottage home to address management problems and by four and half years of age Mary was able to feed herself, help to wash and dress herself, and she was toilet-trained for diurnal bladder control although she still wet the bed regularly.

Some time during the next two years Mary was placed into a foster home with exceptionally good foster parents. She was reassessed psychologically at seven years of age, by which time she was attending a special school for deaf children. At this time she appeared to be happy and to be progressing well within her obvious intellectual limitations. Psychometric reassessment at this time confirmed the earlier impression that Mary was moderately intellectually disabled, with an IQ score of just below 50. It was also felt that she displayed several autistic features, although these were not sufficient in number or severity for her to be diagnosed as an autistic child.

By this time also Mary was fully continent at night as well as during the day. She then remained continent until she was about twelve years of age, when she developed a kidney infection which was accompanied by regression to regular bedwetting. An initial attempt to manage her bedwetting by medical staff treating the kidney infection centred on medication (imipramine, 75 mg at night), which reduced the frequency of bedwetting accidents to two or three per week. However, this treatment never completely arrested her symptoms. Thereafter she remained on medication intermittently for about the next four years, because her medical adviser felt that there was some advantage in two or three wet beds per week as opposed to wetting every night. In addition, the medical staff involved considered that, because of her multiple handicaps, she would not be responsive to forms of therapy that required more of her than simply swallowing pills.

By the time that she had reached 16 years of age it was decided to attempt to treat Mary's bedwetting with a bed-pad and alarm programme at the same hospital, with appropriate modifications to the alarm because of her hearing impairment. The equipment used was the same as that to be described below for treating Paul, another deaf child. Thus, the urine-detector pad was connected to a powerful strobo-scopic light instead of to the usual auditory signal box, but also to a standard buzzer, which was triggered simultaneously in response to wetting accidents and was placed in the foster parents' room. The light was positioned near the bed and directed at Mary's face so that, once triggered by a bedwetting accident, it flashed continuously until turned off. Apart from this specialized equipment, the treatment method

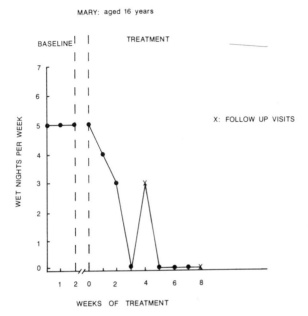

Figure 3.19 Record of Mary's treatment.

followed with Mary was based on the urine-alarm procedure combined with the waking schedule, as described in Chapter 2 for the Dry-Bed Training programme.

Extra care was taken by the therapist when explaining the procedure to Mary but, even so, there was still considerable doubt that she had fully understood what was to follow and what was expected of her. It was thought that, because of the unique set of difficulties presented by Mary, closer than usual therapist supervision and support would be required and arrangements were therefore made for telephone contact with Mary and her foster parents on a regular weekly basis, in addition to the proposed monthly personal visits that they would make to the clinic. As is standard in any of our cases, Mary and her foster parents were invited to contact the therapist at any time if problems arose.

As can be seen from Mary's progress record (Figure 3.19), these apprehensions about possible difficulties were quite unnecessary. When taken off medication in order to establish a baseline for enuresis, Mary's bedwetting frequency increased to approximately five wet nights per week but after the introduction of the urine-alarm device she wet the bed on only eight occasions before reaching the dryness criterion of 21 consecutive dry nights. The time taken from the commencement of treatment to her last wet night was 30 days. Follow-up over the next two years after the termination of treatment confirmed that Mary did not suffer any significant relapse in her bedwetting. Although occasional isolated incidents were reported, no further treatment was necessary.

It is difficult to account for the relative ease with which this 16-year-old girl who was profoundly deaf, intellectually disabled, and who had a visual impairment and early social and emotional deprivation, was trained for nocturnal bladder control. In the event, despite contingency plans, input from the therapist was no greater than for more straightforward cases, these plans not being implemented because they were not required. Certainly the response of the foster parents was excellent; they complied with all instructions for treatment, following the programme to the letter. In retrospect, one is reminded that developing insights into the cause of a bed-wetting problem is not always necessary to effect a cure. Simply ensuring that the appropriate conditioning occurs appears to be the major theraputic agent. Furthermore, Mary's case confirms that the stroboscopic light described above seems to serve as a very effective means for arousing enuretic children with a hearing impairment.

3.14 Treating a very young child

It is not uncommon for medical practitioners to advise parents of enuretic children that no treatment is warranted until the child is at least seven years of age, and often the advice would be to wait until about ten years of age. Moreover, a significant number of medical practitioners hold the belief that, even at ten years and beyond, no treatment at all is to be recommended, based on the observation that children tend to outgrow bedwetting, a generalization which is obviously supported by the age-incidence data. However, we are of the opinion that advice to ignore bedwetting, while highly appropriate for very young children, becomes increasingly inappropriate for older children. Indeed, it is our observation that delaying treatment beyond about five to seven years of age may lead to more significant psychological problems.

There are several reasons for our adopting this position. First, while there is a consistent trend for the incidence of bedwetting to decline with increasing age, the statistical probability for spontaneously achieving continence over a twelve month period is only about one in five for children between the ages of five and twelve years. Secondly, there is no way of predicting when the spontaneous continence will occur. Thirdly, from the incidence data again, it appears that between 1–2% of the adult population remains nocturnally enuretic, so that one cannot be entirely sure that the young enuretic child will in fact outgrow the problem. Fourthly, the longer that the bedwetting symptoms persist, the greater will be the likelihood that the enuretic child will develop more significant secondary psycho-social problems. At the very least, bedwetting may restrict the child's social movements (e.g. attendance at school camps, or staying overnight with friends) but one also runs the risk of damaging the child's self-confidence and self-esteem and heightening tensions within the family if the problem is allowed to continue without treatment. Fifthly, given that treatment based on the urine-alarm procedure is highly effective in arresting bedwetting in the vast majority of cases, and it is a non-invasive and completely safe procedure, it could be argued that there is little to be lost and much to be gained by treating the problem early.

We are of the opinion that children as young as five years can be treated effectively with the urine-alarm device. Of course, much depends on the individual child's level of maturity at this age. Indeed, we have successfully treated children as young as four years, though the permanent success rate at this age is in the order of 50%, compared with the 80–90% success rate that one can expect with older children. None the less, there are sometimes problems associated with treating young bedwetters that do not apply to the same extent with older bedwetters, and these problems may require different management strategies. A major difference that we have noted is that younger bedwetters frequently lack the intrinsic motivation to become dry, and need more direct encouragement and external reinforcement if they are to persist with the programme. The following case of Sam represents a fairly typical experience when treating a very young bedwetter.

Sam was four years and four months of age when his parents sought treatment for his bedwetting. His parents were very pleasant and intelligent folk who were keen to give Sam every support in order to help him overcome the problem. The father was a graduate from an agricultural college and he and his wife ran a successful farm. Their second child was a two-year-old girl who had been born with a severe physical disability, and it was partly the problems associated with managing this child that motivated the parents to seek help with Sam's bedwetting. In addition, the mother had recently discovered that she was pregnant for the third time and both parents were therefore keen to have Sam continent at night prior to the arrival of the baby. In short, then, in spite of Sam's young age, the parents were bothered a great deal by his bedwetting and were anxious to tackle the problem immediately.

Sam had been out of nappies during the day by about two years of age. However, night-time control had never been achieved and he had continued to wet the bed on virtually every night. There was a strong family history of enuresis involving the mother and two maternal aunts, all of whom had wet the bed until they were into their early teens. In addition, Sam was described by his mother as being a very deep sleeper. He had been fully investigated from the medical point of view and no underlying physical abnormality had been detected. The parents had already attempted a number of strategies to arrest the problem, such as lifting during the night, fluid restriction prior to bedtime, and various systems of rewarding dry nights, but all without success. They felt that they had reached a point where professional intervention was necessary but they were, at the same time, worried that they might now be over-reacting to Sam's bedwetting because of these other demands within the family, and that such over-reaction might only make the problem worse.

Sam impressed during the assessment interview as being an alert, active, rough-and-tumble type of child. He appeared to have little appreciation of the reason for attending the interview; he was aware that he wet the bed and that this worried his parents but he seemed not to be bothered much by the problem himself. He was much more interested in playing with the toys in the consulting room than in participating in any discussion about his bedwetting. It was decided to go ahead with the bed-pad and alarm programme with Sam, despite his young age, mainly because of the parents' concern to be rid of an annoying burden on top of the significant demands of having a physically disabled infant and the expected arrival of a third child. In addition, since Sam was able to demonstrate that he already had excellent diurnal bladder control and because he had actually experienced occasional dry nights, it was considered that he had the potential to respond to the standard conditioning procedure.

After establishing a baseline wetting frequency over a period of two weeks, as already described for other cases included here, the treatment programme began. This involved the bed-pad and alarm device, with it being emphasized to Sam's parents that they must ensure that Sam was always awakened in response to bedwetting accidents, taken to the toilet in order to finish voiding and that he then assist the parents to dry the pad and replace the soiled draw sheet before returning to sleep. Because of Sam's age it was expected that the parents would need to take an active role in this process and this they were willing to do. Two sets of records were kept, one by the parents and one by Sam. The parents kept the more comprehensive record sheet, as described earlier, and Sam drew up a calendar with the therapist on which he was to place a sticker for each dry night. It was explained to Sam that these stickers could be converted into some more tangible reward (e.g. a small toy or treat), depending on his progress. A time for weekly telephone contacts was made and Sam and his parents were to be seen in person throughout at four-weekly intervals.

Sam's progress is summarized in Figure 3.20. It will be seen that his initial progress was very pleasing and he achieved four dry nights in the first week of treatment. In addition, he was waking readily in response to the alarm and co-operating with the requirements that he should go to the toilet and also assist in changing the wet sheet following an accident. He maintained a significantly lowered bedwetting frequency for the next few weeks but it became clear during this time that his improvement had reached a plateau. Over the ensuing months his bedwetting frequency slowly increased, though never returning all the way to the initial baseline level. At the first review session four weeks after the beginning of the treatment programme it was readily apparent that Sam's main interest was in cashing in his reward stickers for a toy car that had been negotiated beforehand. The fact that he had been experiencing dry nights did not appear to give him as much pleasure as the car and he was not particularly interested in discussing his progress. At subsequent follow-up sessions Sam's indifferent attitude towards his progress persisted and the only item of interest to him appeared to be in negotiating his next reward. Hand in hand with this, the parents had become increasingly frustrated and angry with Sam's attitude and they reported that the procedure was not always being followed properly. For example, Sam had begun to turn off the alarm prior to going to sleep without telling them and some bedwetting accidents had therefore occurred, without Sam being wakened. As a consequence, the parents were beginning to lose confidence in the procedure. Attempts were made to counter these difficulties along the way by providing extra support, by scheduling pep talks for Sam and by restructuring the reinforcement schedule but none of these changes met with success and after 24 weeks the programme was terminated.

Sam was reviewed some two years later at the age of six

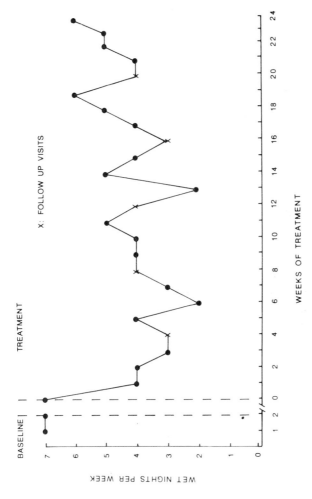

Figure 3.20 Sam's first treatment.

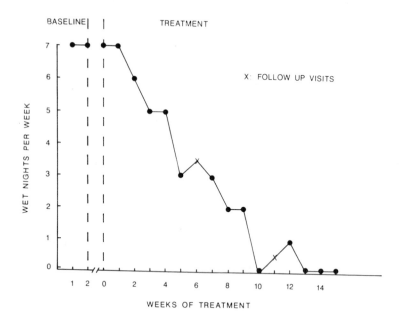

Figure 3.21 Sam's second treatment.

years ten months, at which time he was now wetting the bed on virtually every night. He had not had any formal therapy in the preceding two years and it was readily apparent during the interview that he had matured in general terms during this interval and was now much more motivated to become dry. Thus, it was decided to try again with the same bed-pad and alarm procedure.

Sam's progress the second time around is summarized in Figure 3.21. It can be seen that he made steady progress, culminating in the attainment of the dryness criterion of 21 consecutive dry nights within a treatment period of 15 weeks. The overall experience for the child and his parents was much less stressful on the second occasion, essentially because Sam appeared to now be more intrinsically motivated to become dry. In other words, it now appeared

to matter more to him for personal and social reasons that
he stopped wetting the bed. At follow-up six months later,
he was found to have maintained complete nocturnal
continence.

3.15 Treating a deaf child

Paul was born with a severe hearing impairment, the
aetiology of which was unknown. He first came to the attention of a clinical psychologist at a large metropolitan hospital
when he was referred for routine developmental assessment
at 22 months of age. His abilities were highly variable, with
predictably low scores on items involving speech and
language, but he had advanced visual–motor skills and form
perception. It was concluded that his overall intelligence was
at least average and plans were prepared for him to
experience special early kindergarten training from two-and-
a-half years of age. He had been fitted with hearing aids but
disliked wearing the aids and removed them whenever he
could. This problem was dealt with successfully by a standard behaviour modification procedure.

Paul's progress was monitored over the next few years,
mainly from the point of view of setting up the most appropriate educational programme. By the time that he was five
years of age it had become apparent that he was severely
deaf, even with the use of hearing aids. However, his non-
verbal mental development was now found to be advanced
for his age.

After Paul started school in a special education facility for
deaf children, his contact with the psychology section at the
hospital gradually became more sporadic. When reviewed at
twelve years of age, he was found to be a friendly, co-
operative boy who appeared to have achieved a high level of
social adjustment and academic performance in spite of his
hearing impairment. By this time he wore a special micro-
phone system to boost his hearing aid but, even with this
assistance, he had a severe hearing loss. In the course of this
latter review it was learned that for the first time that Paul

was a regular bedwetter. He was a primary enuretic but this problem had not previously come to attention because it had been overshadowed by the difficulties associated with his hearing. Further questioning established that he had occasionally wet himself during the day-time until eight years of age, when this problem had been resolved spontaneously. The family history was significant, in that his father and a paternal uncle had also been bedwetters as children. Unlike most bedwetters, Paul was reported by his parents as being a light sleeper.

The family had made cursory attempts in the past to curb Paul's bedwetting but had met with little success. Specifically, he had been treated with medication (imipramine) for a brief period and his parents had also attempted to restrict his fluids and had tried various reward systems. Otherwise they had not made much of a fuss about Paul's bedwetting and in the light of the father's experience they had believed that Paul would eventually outgrow the problem. The turning point came, however, when Paul started to demonstrate embarrassment and annoyance with his bedwetting, whereas beforehand it had seemed hardly to bother him at all.

Further psychological assessment, including family dynamics and socio-emotional adjustment, together with medical investigations, revealed no significant problems. It was decided to implement a conditioning treatment programme but the obvious problem was how to develop an alternative to the usual auditory signal in order to awaken Paul in response to wetting accidents. This was achieved by connecting a powerful stroboscopic light which flashed continuously until it was turned off, to the standard urine detector pad, in place of the usual buzzer. In addition, an extension speaker which delivered the usual auditory signal was placed in the parents' bedroom. This was triggered at the same time as the stroboscopic light and was used to summon one of the parents to check whether Paul had been aroused and had completed the required steps of toileting and remaking the bed.

Paul's progress is summarized in Figure 3.22. Altogether he recorded 48 wetting accidents before his symptoms were

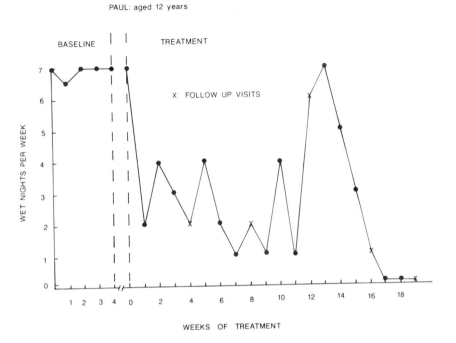

Figure 3.22 Record of Paul's treatment.

arrested and the duration of treatment to the last wet night was about 17 weeks. This was therefore about five to seven weeks longer than the average treatment time for more straightforward cases using the conventional auditory alarm but the outcome was, none the less, an extremely pleasing one. Interestingly, there were only a few occasions when the parents had to wake Paul. The stroboscopic light was found to be highly effective on its own right from the outset. Follow-up contacts with Paul at three, six and twelve months revealed that he had not shown any signs of relapse.

We have subsequently treated four deaf children in a similar manner, obtaining results commensurate with those obtained with Paul. We do not know whether the type of equipment used to treat Paul is commercially available and, in Paul's case, all equipment was designed and constructed by technical staff at the hospital involved. *

It would be possible to develop alternative signals to arouse deaf children who wet the bed. One limitation of the stroboscopic light is that its effectiveness becomes limited if it is not shining directly on the child's face during sleep. Since a child will obviously move around a great deal during the course of a night's sleep, his/her face may be turned away from the light at the time that a bedwetting accident occurs. Although this did not appear to matter in the long run with Paul or the other four deaf children referred to here, it has nevertheless been the case that all of these children have taken longer to cure than usual, and in some instances the stroboscopic procedure has been dependent on the back-up of parents. We suggest that an alternative waking signal worthy of further research and development would be a vibrating device in the form of a mat placed on top of the child's pillow or, alternatively, a vibrator which could be attached to the child's body, e.g. in the form of a wrist-watch device.

3.16 Treating a child with neuropathic bladder impairment

Trudy was born with spina bifida. This condition is a congenital malformation of the vertebral column, in which the posterior bony arch of one or more vertebrae is deficient. In the more common and most serious form of spina bifida (termed myelomeningocele) this bony defect is accompanied by a malformation of the lower end of the spinal cord. Another effect of spina bifida can be the disturbance of the flow of cerebrospinal fluid leading to the development of hydrocephalus. This condition is present in about 90% of cases of myelomeningocele. Hydrocephalus, if significant

* Further details about the lighting system devised to treat Paul can be obtained from the Electronics Department, Adelaide Children's Hospital Incorporated, North Adelaide, South Australia, 5006.

enough, is usually treated surgically within the first few days of life and, while this is a very effective procedure, hydrocephalus can effect the child's intellectual status. Malformation of the spinal cord results in varying degrees of paralysis of the lower limbs – sometimes none at all, sometimes of such severity that walking is impossible. In addition, there is usually some degree of paralysis of the nerves controlling the bladder and bowels, the extent depending on the severity of the damage to the spinal cord.

In Trudy's case, the extent of her disability arising from her spinal bifida was mild. Thus, she was able to walk without difficulty, she was of normal intelligence, she developed bowel control, and ultimately, as will be seen, she was able to develop effective bladder control. None the less, she suffered a mild degree of paralysis of the nerves governing bladder function and hence had the condition known as neuropathic bladder. In mild cases this condition is difficult to diagnose, but Trudy's condition was established by investigations which showed her to have a larger and more flaccid bladder than normal, which she was unable to empty completely of urine.

As a consequence of her neuropathic bladder, Trudy was still frequently wet during the day by the time she started school. However, by about ten years of age she had developed complete urinary continence during the day-time, though she continued to wet the bed regularly and her diurnal bladder control was upset intermittently by urinary tract infections. At twelve years of age, she enquired about the possibility of treatment for her bedwetting from the enuresis clinic at a large metropolitan hospital. By this time, in addition to being reliably dry during the day, she had managed to achieve three to four dry nights per week, due largely to her self-initiated practice of waking during the night for toileting. After consultation with the appropriate medical specialists at the spina bifida clinic, it was felt that Trudy had the neurological competence to warrant an attempt to treat her by the standard bed-pad and alarm method. At this time it was assumed that, like the majority of spina bifida children, she would always be troubled by some small degree of urinary incontinence.

Trudy's family circumstances are also worthy of comment. Her mother had very significant personality problems, necessitating frequent hospital admissions and ongoing psychiatric care. Her father was employed in a semi-skilled occupation. At the commencement of her treatment, both parents were living at home (she was an only child) and, while each parent was concerned about Trudy's welfare, it was apparent that there was a very high degree of marital tension in the home and that the bulk of the responsibility for maintaining the treatment programme would rest firmly on Trudy's shoulders. Indeed, throughout treatment, Trudy took full responsibility for every aspect of the programme, including the washing of her own sheets and soiled bedding. The parents were encouraged to provide support and positive reinforcement but in reality their contribution was limited by the domestic tension and the mother's illness.

Trudy's progress is summarized in Figure 3.23. It can be seen that she responded very rapidly to the bed-pad and alarm programme. Indeed, she recorded only six wet nights prior to reaching the dryness criterion and the time taken to her last wet night was only 13 days. Trudy has been followed up for eight years since this treatment. She maintained urinary continence during both the day and night, with only rare accidents, for five years after treatment. However, when 17 years of age, she was hospitalized for treatment of a urinary tract infection. At that time she reported that she was finding it difficult to void and she appeared to have the sensation of incomplete bladder emptying. A programme of intermittent catheterization was used to empty her bladder and after several days on this procedure she was again able to void normally and the catheterization procedure was discontinued.

A year later she was again admitted to hospital, this time because of persistent abdominal pain and difficulty with voiding. Ultrasound examination showed that she had ovarian cysts and also confirmed early evidence of a large neuropathic bladder. She again commenced intermittent catheterization, which was effective in emptying her bladder and enabled her to return to normal spontaneous voiding.

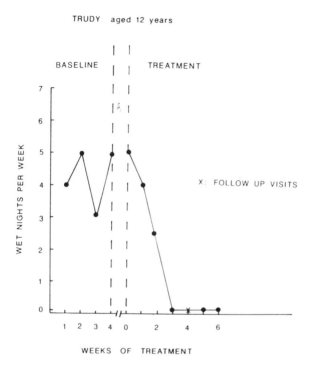

Figure 3.23 Record of Trudy's treatment.

Since there were no significant symptoms from the ovarian cyst she was discharged after a few days and her diurnal and nocturnal bladder control has been normal since that time.

This is a case of particular significance because the expectation of successfully treating a bedwetter with known neuropathic bladder ordinarily would be very low. Presumably, Trudy had sufficient neurological competence remaining to enable her to establish bladder control and, in more severe cases, no amount of training could be effective. The case also raises interesting questions in respect of the interface between the roles of neurological maturation (and/or competence) and conditioning in the establishment of bladder control. Clearly both processes are involved although the actual dynamics are not yet fully understood. It is conceivable, however, that someone in Trudy's situation, because of her disability would not have the same expectations placed on him/her to establish bladder control and therefore not be subjected to the same degree of social conditioning that takes place in the ordinary course of toilet training. It is conceivable also that other people with 'borderline' neurological impairment resulting in urinary incontinence (e.g. other mild cases of spina bifida, individuals with low spinal lesions caused by trauma, or aged people), could be helped by appropriate conditioning methods.

3.17 Comments on three cases of bedwetting in adulthood

Surveys of the incidence of bedwetting indicate that possibly 1–2% of adults are nocturnally enuretic. It is likely that a high proportion of this group would be intellectually disabled to some degree, or would be found on urodynamic examination of the lower urinary tract to have unstable bladders caused by uncontrolled contractive activity of the detrusor muscle. Such cases would commonly also involve diurnal enuresis. These groups aside, however, there are certainly also significant numbers of normal, healthy adults in the community who regularly wet the bed.

The present authors have encountered ten such adult bedwetters in the course of treating almost 2000 nocturnally enuretic children and adolescents since 1975. One of the striking features of this group of adult bedwetters is that none has chosen to pursue treatment. Although research data on adult bedwetters are limited, there are studies to suggest that adults, like children, respond well to the bed-pad and alarm programme. In light of our experience, however, it seems possible that the psychological dynamics associated with many adult bedwetters may differ in fundamental ways when compared with most enuretic children and these dynamics almost certainly become more complex over time. The following three brief case histories have been chosen to illustrate some experiences in dealing with adult bedwetters.

MARYANNE

The first case history was a 26-year-old woman whom we will call Maryanne. Initial contact with the therapist was made by Maryanne's mother who was highly concerned about her daughter's bedwetting problem and, at this time, Maryanne was unaware of her mother's enquiry. After reassurances from the therapist that other adults wet the bed regularly and that treatment could still be effective, the mother described Maryanne's situation in more detail. Essentially, Maryanne had been a lifelong bedwetter. The problem had resisted all previous treatment attempts including reward systems, waking schedules, an attempt with a bed-pad and alarm programme, and medication. She was an only child and had always displayed an introverted personality, although she had above-average intellectual abilities. From an early age she had preferred to engage herself in music and study rather than more social pastimes. Her mother was unaware of any significant emotional conflicts in Maryanne's life during childhood. She had seemed to reflect the personalities and interests of her parents in general terms, though there was no known family history of enuresis. During adolescence, Maryanne had showed little interest in going out socially and had never had a boyfriend. She had graduated in music with a bachelor degree at university and had subsequently taught piano at the conservatorium and given private tuition from her home. After graduation she moved away from her parent's house, into a home unit where she lived on her own.

Only her parents knew that she still wet the bed and Maryanne became extremely angry when her mother informed her that she had made contact with a therapist. While apparently embarrassed by the problem, Maryanne had shown virtually no interest in seeking treatment since early adolescence. None the less, her mother felt justified in taking the initiative to enquire about treatment because she believed that Maryanne had been held back by her own inhibitions and that achieving nocturnal continence would be in her own best interests. The first task then was to broach the subject with Maryanne in a constructive and positive way. It was suggested that the mother should discuss with Maryanne the telephone conversation that she had had with the therapist, explaining her reasons for taking this initiative and reassuring Maryanne that the chances of effecting a cure were very high. Beyond this it was suggested that it should be left up to Maryanne to take any further steps to seek treatment.

A few weeks later, Maryanne contacted the therapist and arranged an appointment. From the initial assessment interview it was clear that she was a highly intelligent but socially awkward and very defensive young woman. She was passive and uncertain and found it difficult to discuss her enuresis or aspects of her social and domestic life. She did not relate that at the time of the interview she was wetting the bed on approximately three nights each week. She would usually wake immediately after wetting and then get up and change the soiled bedding. Often she was able to recall having a particular dream which seemed to be associated with the bedwetting episodes. The common theme in these dreams was the sensation of voiding but at the same time there was an uneasy awareness that the voiding was inappropriate. For example, she might dream that she had started out by going to the toilet in the normal way but then there might be an abrupt realization that she was voiding in a public place. On some occasions she would sleep throughout the night without waking and discover that the bed was wet the next morning. She explained that she was reluctant to pursue therapy because of her past failures with treatment. The possible reasons for these failures were reviewed and she was reassured that the bed-pad and alarm programme, with appropriate support and supervision, still offered a high likelihood of a cure. However, Maryanne decided against pursuing treatment and nothing more was heard from her after the initial assessment interview.

On the face of it, Maryanne's attitude appears difficult to understand. One can easily appreciate her embarrassment at having to admit to such a problem as a young adult but, once this had been brought into the open and reassurances provided, it seems surprising that Maryanne would not agree to try treatment. It is possible that Maryanne's bedwetting was associated with doubts about her social adequacy and that this helped her to justify her socially isolated lifestyle and in particular to avoid close relationships with men. However, there was no direct evidence for this. In retrospect, it would seem likely that Maryanne was too embarrassed to discuss her bedwetting problem in depth with a male therapist and it is a pity that it did not occur to us to involve a female therapist, as was subsequently done so successfully in the case of Angela (section 3.9).

TONY

Tony attended the initial assessment interview accompanied by his wife who had taken the initiative in arranging the appointment. Tony was 24 years of age, in good physical health and a carpenter by trade. He had a past history of bedwetting until the age of about 16 years. The pattern of his bedwetting had always been sporadic, with an increase in frequency usually associated with periods of stress. For example, while he was still at school the frequency of his bedwetting had usually increased during school examinations. He had not been a good student in academic subjects but had shown a flair for technical subjects. After leaving school, he had entered into an apprenticeship, eventually finding employment as a carpenter. His bedwetting ceased at this time, presumably as a result of his no longer being stressed by subjects with which he had difficulties at school. He had not had any form of therapy for his enuresis, apart from social rewards and punishments implemented by his parents from time to time during his childhood.

After leaving school, Tony wet the bed only very occasionally – perhaps no more than two or three incidents per year. These usually occurred after he had been out the night before and drunk an excessive quantity of alcohol. He had met his wife Rosa when he was eighteen years of age and they had married about five years later, some twelve months prior to our contact. Rosa had been aware of Tony's occasional bedwetting prior to their marriage but these episodes had been regarded as something of a joke. However, six months or so after becoming married, the frequency of Tony's bedwetting increased steadily, to the point where he was wetting the bed almost every night. These incidents resulted in Tony and his wife sleeping in separate beds and a great deal of animosity between them, especially since any attempt on Rosa's part to discuss the problem and encourage Tony to seek help was invariably met with a firm rebuff from him. Eventually, Rosa gave Tony an ultimatum that he either seek treatment for the problem or she would seek a separation in their marriage.

The initial interview was highly emotionally charged. Rosa appeared to be a sensible and caring woman who was very supportive of her husband. Tony was far less confident and was obviously uncomfortable at the interview. The embarrassment he experienced about his bedwetting was dealt with fairly easily but it was readily apparent that there were other fundamental problems within the marital relationship. Reassurances were given about the prospect of arresting the bedwetting with the bed-pad and alarm procedure and it was suggested that this form of therapy be supplemented by marital counselling. The equipment was demonstrated and Rosa re-emphasized her support. However, Tony chose not to pursue any treatment and the therapist was not surprised to learn several weeks later that they had in fact separated.

On reflection, it is quite plausible to regard the resumption of Tony's bedwetting following his marriage as a stress reaction. It was clearly the case that he had a past history of intermittent periods of bedwetting, the onset of which usually coincided with times of stress in his life. The reasons for his rejection of treatment are less clear, however. It is possible that he simply refused to accept direction from his wife. It is also possible that rejection of treatment was a means of forcing a termination to his marriage, within which there clearly were significant problems.

DOROTHY

The third case history is that of a 40-year-old woman named Dorothy who attended an initial assessment interview with her 12-year-old son, Damian, who had been referred for treatment of primary nocturnal enuresis. In the course of this interview Dorothy was asked about whether there was any family history of enuresis, this being a standard part of the assessment protocol. However, when this question was asked there was a slight pause and then both mother and child burst into laughter. Dorothy then quite openly admitted that she still wet the bed regularly and that she had, in fact, wet the night before our meeting. Further questioning revealed that Dorothy had been a regular bedwetter until some time during her teenage years, when she had seemed to outgrow the problem. She had then remained continent, with virtually no regressions at all, until the birth of her fourth child. However, after this delivery she had begun to experience bedwetting incidents at a frequency of approximately one per month. She had subsequently had two further children and following each of these births the bedwetting problem had appeared to become more severe. Thus, at the time of our contact she was wetting the bed on approximately three nights per week. When asked about her reaction to her bedwetting, Dorothy admitted that she was annoyed by having to do extra washing but beyond this it did not bother her at all. She believed that she had a 'weak bladder' and that there was nothing she could do about it. She still shared a bed with her husband and when asked about his reaction to the problem she merely said that he did not seem to mind.

It was suggested to Dorothy that she too would benefit from a trial on the urine-alarm device and this was offered to her immediately following Damian's treatment. Damian proved to be a good candidate for the bed-pad and alarm programme and his symptoms were arrested without difficulty after about ten weeks of treatment. However, Dorothy chose not to pursue the same programme for herself, in spite of Damian's success. She seemed to feel that she was too old for the treatment and simply could not be bothered. There did not appear to be any more subtle or underlying reasons for this attitude. The door was left open for Dorothy to make contact again at any time in the future if she changed her mind but nothing more was heard from her.

4

Directions for future research

The latter half of the twentieth century has seen an enormous increase in world-wide professional interest in the nature of nocturnal enuresis and how this problem might best be corrected. By far, most of the considerable body of literature now available on this topic has been published since 1950 and it is now clear that the treatment of bedwetting forms a major part of the professional activities of large numbers of psychologists and other professionals from a wide range of specializations. Yet despite the progress made in formulating and improving methods for treatment, it must be obvious to any reader of this book that there are many questions in this area for which we are not able to provide satisfactory answers. Undoubtedly, one of these questions must be why the bed-pad and alarm procedure is as effective as it is. It is not known to what extent the alarm serves to condition specific responses to bladder filling, or whether such learning is always best described in terms of passive avoidance, or the extent to which learning is dependent on relative efficacy of social and motivational considerations within the family and broader community setting. However, while these issues are central to a theoretical understanding of the processes involved in the treatment of bedwetting, we have decided to limit our suggestions here to just three areas of immediate practical concern, of which we have become aware both on the basis of our own practical experience and also as a consequence of having recently completed a comprehensive review of research in this field (Bollard and Nettelbeck, in press). These three considerations are, first, the extent to which enuretic children are more difficult to arouse from sleep than nonenuretic children; secondly, the extent of individual differences between enuretic children with respect to a range of bedwetting-related variables and the implications that such differences might have for the application of treatment procedures; and, thirdly, the problem of relapse, with bedwetting resuming at some later time after an initially successful treatment has been effected. We will therefore take each of these areas of concern in turn.

4.1 The sleep-arousal system and enuresis

We have already noted in Chapter 2, that there have been frequent anecdotal reports that children who wet the bed sleep more deeply than do nonenuretic children, and that there is a substantial body of empirical evidence for some kind of an association between enuresis and an impairment of the sleep-arousal system. In addition to these findings, our attention is drawn to the notion of an association between bedwetting and arousal from sleep for essentially two reasons.

First, it is our experience that the majority of the parents who have sought treatment for their children have reported that these children to be very difficult to arouse from sleep prior to treatment; in fact it has typically been the case that these children have been reported to have had a life-long history of deep sleep. Furthermore, most parents with whom we have been involved have reported a tendency for their children to arouse more quickly from sleep as treatment has progressed, and for this change in sleep habits to become habitual after continence had been achieved. Researchers do commonly caution against accepting parents' reports at face value but, while we recognize that parental reports may be biased by the parents' preconceived ideas about the aetiology of enuresis, we are inclined to give credence to such reports. For one thing, we have most frequently found parents' observations of their children's behaviour to be fairly reliable. For another, some of the reasons advanced for rejecting parents' views are patently inaccurate. Thus, it is sometimes claimed that the parents of an enuretic child will not have had much experience with the sleep habits of nonenuretic children – a proposition which our experience and, indeed, common sense would reject. In effect, we believe that it is noteworthy that such parental observations about the sleep characteristics of their children who wet the bed are very frequent.

Secondly, our research into the efficacy of the various components of the Dry-Bed Training procedure has convinced us that the inclusion of the waking schedule from that procedure, together with the standard bed-pad and alarm conditioning procedure, does facilitate response to treatment, perhaps by helping to develop ease of arousability from sleep in the child. However, this assumption has not been tested and further research into the use of waking schedules as adjuvant procedures is necessary. In addition, it may be possible to improve the effectiveness of the Dry-Bed Training waking schedule by staggering the time of the awakenings throughout the night as was done by Young (1964) and Creer and Davis (1975) and/or by the use of the intermittent schedule of awakenings (i.e. waking on some nights but not on others).

In order to explore further the sleep-arousal issue, sleep patterns might be monitored electroencephalographically (EEG) under the following conditions:

1. just prior to and during the act of bedwetting;
2. throughout the course of treatment, comparing the impact of various adjuvant therapies aimed at facilitating arousal from sleep with the effects of the standard conditioning procedure based on the bed-pad and alarm;
3. following the achievement of nocturnal urinary continence;
4. at the time of relapse, should this occur.

EEG monitoring of sleep patterns could be supplemented by measures of arousability from sleep, such as the intensity of the auditory stimulus required to achieve wakefulness, a procedure suggested by Finley (1971). In this way it should be possible to observe whether the development of bladder control is related to changes within the sleep-arousal system and, if so, whether such changes need to be permanent for sustained continence to be achieved. Such observations would also permit the determination of the degree of cortical arousal caused by the alarm which was necessary for the effectiveness of treatment by the standard bed-pad and alarm procedure.

Related issues are whether adjuvant therapies to the bed-pad and alarm procedure do facilitate necessary cortical arousal; and the relative effectiveness of such additional procedures. One of the more obvious possible adjuvant therapies that might be investigated is the use of drugs. Lovibond (1964) has noted that stimulant drugs such as amphetamine sulphate have been used in clinical practice as an accompaniment to the conditioning treatment of enuresis in difficult cases. Young and Turner (1965) found that when drugs that stimulate the central nervous system, like Methedrine and Dexedrine, were administered during conditioning treatment, then this resulted in more rapid initial arrest of bedwetting, although the frequency of relapse was particularly high for subjects to whom Dexedrine had been administered. However, to this time there has been very little systematic study of drug effectiveness as an adjunct to standard conditioning and further research of this kind is warranted.

4.2 Matching particular treatment procedures with the individual needs of the enuretic child

The tendency in research into the treatment of bedwetting has been to develop procedures and to apply these routinely and uniformly to all enuretic children. However, as the various case studies described in Chapter 3 illustrate, in any large group of enuretic children one does find considerable variability in terms of bedwetting frequency, functional bladder capacity, the presence of diurnal symptoms, ease of arousability from sleep, motivation to become dry, willingness to comply with instructions, and so on. Thus, if a single treatment programme is to accommodate these individual differences, it must combine a variety of training strategies. Essentially, this is what has been attempted by

Azrin *et al.* (1973, 1974) when developing the Dry-Bed Training procedure, and research has now shown that this composite treatment 'package' approach is highly successful. A problem with such a comprehensive training programme, however, is that the treatment becomes excessively burdensome. Furthermore, if the full programme is used routinely for all children treated, then some part of the training will be unnecessary for some of the individuals. Our own research in this area has demonstrated that the retention control training and positive practice components of Dry-Bed Training do not effectively advance the rate of progress made by many children treated by this procedure, although we have certainly encountered cases where these training techniques have proved useful.

An alternative and more efficient approach would be to comprehensively assess the enuretic child beforehand, if one were able to do so in terms of characteristics known to influence training outcome, and then to match particular procedures with those training needs. In this way the complexities of treatment might be reduced to a minimum. Of course, to this time it has not proved possible to specify such characteristics in any detail, although considerations like functional bladder capacity, ease of arousability from sleep and motivation to become dry do appear to provide useful leads. On the basis of our own research (e.g. Bollard and Nettelbeck, 1982) we are satisfied that the standard bed-pad and alarm procedure provides the most suitable 'core' treatment for bedwetting. However, comprehensive assessment prior to treatment could indicate that additional forms of therapy would be beneficial in some cases. For example, where a child's functional bladder capacity appeared to be low (suggested, for example, by parents' reports), then capacity could be measured by the water load technique described in section 2.1; and if this test confirmed the earlier judgement, then the conditioning procedure could be supplemented by daily retention control training. Similarly, ease of arousability from sleep could be assessed before treatment by having the parent measure the degree of intensity of an auditory stimulus necessary to awaken the child from sleep, or by timing the interval between presentation of an auditory stimulus and the child awakening. It might not even be necessary to measure arousability from sleep beforehand, but rather it might be possible to make this assessment based on the child's response to the bed-pad and alarm during the first few days of treatment. In any case, if the child was particularly difficult to arouse from sleep, the standard conditioning procedure could be supplemented by an adjuvant therapy such as a nightly waking schedule or even an appropriate drug as discussed in section 2.4. Indeed, as we have already emphasized elsewhere in Chapter 2, a combination of the standard bed-pad and alarm procedure with the waking schedule from Dry-Bed Training is sufficient to meet the needs of the vast majority of childhood bedwetters. If poor motivation was a characteristic of the child before treatment, then the standard alarm programme could be supplemented by more intensive differential reinforcement for wet or dry nights.

Furthermore, as pointed out by Doleys and Ciminero (1976), a thorough behavioural history may also uncover other behaviours, such as fear of the dark and toilet phobia, that may be related functionally to bedwetting, and which should be eliminated prior to commencing treatment of the bedwetting itself. Information relating to parental attitudes and the ability of parents to conduct the training would also be worthwhile.

4.3 The problem of relapse

In the clinical setting, there are at least two issues of practical concern which arise as a consequence of a relapse following an initially successful treatment based on the bed-pad with alarm procedure. One issue is the total amount of time required to eradicate the bedwetting – i.e. the time to achieve an initial arrest of bedwetting, together with any additional time for the treatment of the relapse. This time defines the duration for which equipment will be committed to the treatment of the individual case, a very important consideration, especially when urine-alarm devices are in short supply. The other problem associated with relapse concerns the possibility that parents and children will become disillusioned with the training programme following relapse, and therefore be less motivated to seek re-treatment.

In addressing this first issue, one could adopt the view that the possibility of relapse is a shortcoming of conditioning treatments and that, at least in many cases, further therapy will inevitably be required. An implication of this position is that a major aim of treatment should be to achieve initial dryness as quickly as possible, thereby minimizing the total time for alarm usage. From this viewpoint, Dry-Bed Training with its additional procedures has some advantage over the standard dry-pad and alarm method which does not involve those procedures. Thus an initial arrest in bedwetting is reached more quickly on average when following the full Dry-Bed Training routine that with the standard procedure, and there is little difference between the two methods in terms of either the rate of subsequent relapse or the successful retreatment of renewed bedwetting. On the other hand, as has been noted in Chapter 2, Dry-Bed Training does have a number of practical problems as a result of the demanding procedures included and these do limit its large-scale application. Furthermore, simply minimizing the total time for alarm-usage does not overcome the significant problem that some parents and children will regard a relapse as a failure, become disillusioned with the programme and therefore not seek re-treatment. Thus, there is still a need to develop a treatment that arrests bedwetting quickly but that also results in a lower rate of relapse.

A starting point might be to incorporate an intermittent schedule of alarm presentation and/or to introduce over-learning trials into the bed-pad with alarm procedure, accompanied by the waking schedule from Dry-Bed Training. Any decline in relapse rate resulting from these procedures would have to weighed up against any increase in the initial treatment time. A second possibility strategy for reducing the relapse problem could be the combination of retention control training with the urine-alarm and waking procedure.

The only factor found reliably to predict proneness to relapse following conditioning treatment is a child's history of daytime wetting difficulties. These problems of diurnal urgency, frequency and wetting accidents are most likely explained by lower than normal levels of functional bladder capacity. Overall, the data from studies which have employed retention control training suggest that, while such training is of limited value in arresting bedwetting, it can be quite effective in increasing functional bladder capacity. Thus, retention control training when used in conjunction with the urine-alarm device may result in a more permanent dryness response. It is likely that retention control training would need to be practised daily over several months in order for it to have a therapeutic effect and this would doubtless increase the demands of the method of treatment. Thus, to avoid placing unnecessary demands on children not likely to benefit from retention control training, this would only be introduced for those children who were found to have severely low functional bladder capacities, as indicated by a pre-treatment water load test and/or a history of diurnal micturitional difficulty. In the meantime, until an effective method for significantly reducing the rate of relapse following treatment based on the bed-pad and alarm is achieved, it would seem desirable to warn parents and children beforehand that there is a high likelihood of another period on the alarm being necessary at some time in the future in order to achieve a complete cure.

References

American Psychiatric Association (1980) *Diagnostic and Statistical Manual of Mental Disorders*. (3rd edition), APA, Washington, DC.

Azrin, N.H. and Foxx, R.M. (1974) *Toilet Training in Less Than a Day*. Simon and Schuster, New York.

Azrin, N.H., Sneed, T.J. and Foxx, R.M. (1973) Dry bed: A rapid method of eliminating bedwetting (enuresis) of the retarded. *Behaviour Research and Therapy*, **11**, 427–34.

Azrin, N.H., Sneed, T.J. and Foxx, R.M. (1974) Dry-bed training: Rapid elimination of childhood enuresis. *Behaviour Research and Therapy*, , **12**, 147–56.

Bakwin, H. (1971) Enuresis in twins. *American Journal of Diseases in Children*, **121**, 222–5.

Baller, W.R. (1975) *Bed-wetting: Origins and Treatment*. Pergamon Press, New York.

Bettison, S. (1979) Toilet training. In *Children's Problems*. (eds M. Griffin and A. Hudson), Circus Books, Melbourne.

Bettison, S. (1986) Behavioral approaches to toilet training for retarded persons. In *International Review of Research in Mental Retardation*. Vol. 14, (eds N.R. Ellis and N.W. Bray), Academic Press, New York, pp. 319–50.

Bjornsson, S. (1973) Enuresis in childhood: its incidence and associations with intelligence, emotional disorder, and some social and educational variables. *Scandanavian Journal of Educational Research*, **17**, 63–82.

Blackwell, B. and Currah, J. (1973) The pharmacology of enuresis. In *Bladder Control and Enuresis*. (eds I. Kolvin, R.C. MacKeith and S.R. Meadow), Lippincott, Philadelphia, pp. 231–51.

Bollard, J and Nettelbeck, T. (1981) A comparison of Dry-Bed Training and standard urine-alarm conditioning treatment of childhood bedwetting. *Behaviour Research and Therapy*, **19**, 215–26.

Bollard, J. and Nettelbeck, T. (1982) A component analysis of Dry-Bed Training for treatment of bedwetting. *Behaviour Research and Therapy*, **20**, 383–90.

Bollard, J. and Nettelbeck, T. (in press) The behavioral management of nocturnal enuresis. In *International Perspectives in Behavioral Medicine*. Volume II, (eds D.G. Byrne and G.R. Caddy), Ablex, Norwood, NJ.

Broughton, R.F. (1968) Sleep disorders: disorders of arousal? *Science*, **159**, 1070–8.

Butler, R.J. (1987) *Nocturnal Enuresis: Psychological Perspectives*. IOP Publishing (Wright), Bristol.

Choice (1977) Bedwetting alarms. *Choice*, September, 322–5.

Collins, R.W. (1973) Importance of the bladder–cue buzzer contingency in the conditioning treatment of enuresis. *Journal of Abnormal Psychology*, **82**, 299–308.

Coote, M.A. (1965) Apparatus for conditioning treatment of enuresis. *Behaviour Research and Therapy*, **2**, 233–8.

Creer, T.L. and Davis, M.H. (1975) Using a staggered waking procedure with enuretic children in an institutional setting. *Journal of Behavior Therapy and Experimental Psychiatry*, **6**, 23–5.

De Jonge, G.A. (1973) Epidemiology of enuresis: a survey of the literature. In *Bladder Control and Enuresis*. (eds I. Kolvin, R.C. MacKeith, and S.R. Meadow), Lippincott, Philadelphia, pp. 39–46.

De Leon, G. and Mandell, W. (1966) A comparison of conditioning and psychotherapy in the treatment of functional enuresis. *Journal of Clinical Psychology*, **22**, 326–30.

De Perri, R. and Meduri, M. (1972) L'enuresi notturna: ulteriori elementi in tema di diagnostica strumentale. *Acta Neuroligica Napoli*, **27**, 22–7.

Dische, S., Yule, W., Corbett, J. and Hand, D. (1983) Childhood nocturnal enuresis: factors associated with outcome of treatment with an enuresis alarm. *Developmental Medicine and Child Neurology*, **25**, 67–80.

Doleys, D.M. (1977) Behavioral treatments for nocturnal enuresis in children: A review of the recent literature. *Psychological Bulletin*, **84**, 30–54.

Doleys, D.M. and Ciminero, A.R. (1976) Childhood enuresis: considerations in treatment. *Journal of Pediatric Psychology*, **4**, 21–3.

Essen, J. and Peckham, C. (1976) Nocturnal enuresis in childhood. *Developmental Medicine and Child Neurology*, **18**, 577–89.

Finley, W.W. (1971) An EEG study of the sleep of enuretics at three age levels. *Clinical Electroencephalography*, **2**, 35–9.

Glicklich, L.B. (1951) An historical account of enuresis. *Pediatrics*, **8**, 859.

Goel, K.M., Thomson, R.B., Gibb, E.M. and McAinsh, T.F. (1984) Evaluation of nine different types of enuresis alarms. *Archives of Disease in Childhood*, **59**, 748–53.

Greaves, M.W. (1969) Hazards of enuresis alarm. *Archives of Disease in Children*, **44**, 285–6.

Hunt, G., Long, J. and Long, J. (Undated) *Nocturnal Enuresis: Management Systems and Equipment Evaluation*. Unpublished research report, Oxford Regional Health Authority.

Johnson, S.B. (1980) Enuresis. In *Clinical Behavior Therapy and Behavior Modification*, Volume 1, (ed. R.D. Daitzman), Garland STPM Press, New York, pp. 81–142.

Jureidini, K. (1982) Enuresis: Helping the patients and parents. *Patient Management*, December, pp. 25–8.

Kolvin, I., MacKeith, R.C. and Meadow, S.R. (eds) (1973) *Bladder Control and Enuresis*, Lippincott, Philadelphia.

Kolvin, I. and Taunch, J. (1973) A dual theory of nocturnal enuresis. In *Bladder Control and Enuresis*. (eds I. Kolvin, R.C. MacKeith and S.R. Meadow), Lippincott, Philadelphia, pp. 156–72.

Lovibond, S.H. (1964) *Conditioning and Enuresis*. Pergamon Press, Oxford.

MacKeith, R., Meadow, R. and Turner, R.K. (1973) How children become dry. In *Bladder Control and Enuresis*. (eds I. Kolvin, R.C. MacKeith and S.R. Meadow), Lippincott, Philadelphia, pp. 3–21.

Mandelstam, D. (ed.) (1986) *Incontinence and its Management*. 2nd edition, Croom Helm, London.

McKendry, J.B.J. and Stewart, D.A. (1974) Enuresis. *Pediatric Clinics of North America*, **21**, 1019–28.

Morgan, R.T.T. (1978) Relapse and therapeutic response in the conditioning treatment of enuresis: A review of recent findings on intermittent reinforcement, overlearning and stimulus intensity. *Behaviour Research and Therapy*, **16**, 273–9.

Mountjoy, P.T., Ruben, D.H. and Bradford, T.S. (1984) Recent technological advancements in the treatment of enuresis. *Behavior Modification*, **8**, 291–315.

Mowrer, O.H. and Mowrer, W.M. (1938) Enuresis: a method for its study and treatment. *American Journal of Orthopsychiatry*, **8**, 436–59.

Muellner, S.R. (1960a) Development of urinary control in children. *Journal of the American Medical Association*, **172**, 1256–61.

Muellner, S.R. (1960b) Development of urinary control in children. A new concept in cause, prevention and treatment in primary enuresis. *Journal of Urology*, **84**, 714–16.

Neal, B.W. and Coote, M.A. (1969) Hazards of enuresis alarm. *Archives of Disease of Children*, **44**, 651.

Oppel, W.C., Harper, P.A. and Rider, R.V. (1968) The age of attaining bladder control. *Pediatrics*, **42**, 614.

Pfaundler, M. (1904) Demonstration eines apparatus zur selstätigen stattgehabter Bettnäsung. *Verhandlungen der Gesellschaft für Kinderheilkunde*, **21**, 219.

Pfeiffer, D.G. and Lloyd, D.T. (1978) Enuresis alarm innovations. *Monitor-Proceedings of the I.R.E.E., Australia*, September/October, pp. 148–50.

Rutter, M., Yule, W. and Graham, P. (1973) Enuresis and behavioral deviance: some epidemiological considerations. In *Bladder Control and Enuresis*. (eds I. Kolvin, R.C. MacKeith and S.R. Meadow), Lippincott, Philadelphia, pp. 137–50.

Sacks, S., De Leon, G. and Blackman, S. (1974) Psychological changes associated with conditioning functional enuresis. *Journal of Clinical Psychology*, **30**, 271–6.

Schaefer, C.E. (1979) *Childhood Encopresis and Enuresis: Causes and Therapy*. Van Nostrand Reinhold, New York.

Shaffer, D. (1973) The association between enuresis and emotional disorder: A review of the literature. In *Bladder Control and Enuresis*. (eds I. Kolvin, R.C. MacKeith and S.R. Meadow), Lippincott, Philadelphia, pp. 118–36.

Shaffer, D. (1980) The development of bladder control. In *Scientific Foundations of Developmental Psychiatry*. (ed. M. Rutter), William Heinemann, London.

Smith, P.S. and Smith, L.J. (1987) *Continence and Incontinence: Psychological Approaches to Development and Treatment*. Croom Helm, London.

Sorotzkin, B. (1984) Nocturnal enuresis: current perspectives. *Clinical Psychology Review*, **4**, 293–316.

Taylor, P.D. and Turner, R.K. (1975) A clinical trial of continuous, intermittent and overlearning 'bell-and-pad' treatments for nocturnal enuresis. *Behaviour Research and Therapy*, **2**, 567–74.

Verhulst, F.C., van der Lee, J.H., Akkerhuis, G.W., Sanders-Woudstray, G.W., Timmer, F.C. and Donkhorst, I.D. (1985) The prevalence of nocturnal enuresis: do DSMIII Criteria need to be changed? A brief research report. *Journal of Child Psychology and Psychiatry*, **26**, 989–93.

Weir, K. (1982) Night and day wetting among a population of three-year-olds. *Developmental Medicine and Child Neurology*, **24**, 479–84.

Werry, J.S. and Cohrssen, J. (1965) Enuresis: an etiologic and therapeutic study. *Journal of Pediatrics*, **67**, 423–31.

Yates, A.J. (1975) *Theory and Practice in Behavior Therapy*. Wiley, New York.

Young, G.C. (1964) A 'staggered-awakening' procedure in the treatment of enuresis. *Medical Officer*, **111**, 142–3.

Young, G.C. and Morgan, R.T.T. (1972) Childhood enuresis: termination of treatment by parents. *Community Medicine*, **129**, 247–50.

Young, G.C. and Turner, R.K. (1965) CNS stimulant drugs and conditioning of nocturnal enuresis. *Behaviour Research and Therapy*, **3**, 93–101.

Appendix

Instructions for use of the urine-alarm device

The bedwetting alarm is run on a large torch battery and is electrically quite harmless even if the child touches contacts. If the alarm is to work properly, however, you must follow the instructions carefully.

STEP 1

Place the alarm unit (buzzer) in a firm position near to the head of the bed. It is important to have the unit as near as is practicable to the child's ear but beyond reach, so that the child has to get out of bed in order to switch off the alarm when it is triggered. Do not put the unit on a soft surface as this muffles the sound of the alarm.

STEP 2

Make up the bed in this order:

(a) rubber sheet to protect mattress;
(b) normal sheet on top of the waterproof covering;
(c) electrode pad positioned on the bed so that it covers the area where the child will wet when sleeping in the usual position; i.e. place the pad underneath the child's buttocks. When a single pad system is used it is important to make sure that the wire electrode strips are pointing upwards. Where the alarm system uses two pads, a small flannelette sheet is placed between the two pads. This sheet should not contain any holes and should extend about 20 cm (8 inches) beyond the perimeter of the pads;

(d)   a draw sheet is placed over the pad/s in order to secure it in the correct position and to ensure that the child does not sleep directly on the electrode pad;

(e)   normal bedding on top of the child.

STEP 3

Connect the urine detector pad to the alarm unit according to the specifications of the particular equipment being used. For single pad units, the connecting wire is usually permanently attached to the pad and is connected to the alarm unit by inserting one or two plugs into designated holes. Where the alarm system uses two pads, each pad is attached to the alarm unit by a lead with press-stud or crocodile-clip connections. Where the two pads are made from wire meshing, the crocodile-clips must pass beyond the peripheral binding around the pads and make contact with the mesh, and the clips on the two mats must not lie on top of each other.

STEP 4

Turn the alarm switch 'on'. This means that the alarm is now ready. If it goes off at this time then the alarm is faulty and the therapist should be notified before proceeding further with treatment.

STEP 5

The child should sleep without pyjama pants. If the child objects to this, try removing them after he/she is asleep. If there are further objections, a suitable compromise is to allow the child to wear thin summer pyjamas.

STEP 6

When the alarm goes off it means that the child has wet the bed. The procedure that follows bedwetting is set out below.

(a) The child turns off the alarm. (If the child does not wake to the alarm then a parent should shake the child gently until he/she wakes up.)

(b) The child goes to the toilet to finish urinating.

(c) The child changes into clean pyjamas, removes the wet draw sheet from the bed, wipes the rubber pad dry and then deposits the wet sheet in the laundry.

(d) The child remakes the bed (with parental assistance if necessary), as described in Step 2.

(e) The child switches the bedwetting alarm on again.

(f) The child returns to sleep.

CLEANING THE PAD

The pad is sterilized before it is loaned to parents, and no cleaning agent should be used on it. Before returning it, however, please wipe it over with warm water and soap. After drying it, please roll it up, or pack it away according to the instructions printed on the underside of the pad.

ALARM NOT WORKING PROPERLY

If the alarm does not sound following a bedwetting accident, or if it sounds without a bedwetting accident having occurred, contact the therapist as quickly as possible.

Author index

Subject index